MAKING ROOM FOR MADNESS IN MENTAL HEALTH

MAKING ROOM FOR MADNESS IN MENTAL HEALTH

The Psychoanalytic Understanding
of Psychotic Communication

Marcus Evans

Foreword by
Edna O'Shaughnessy

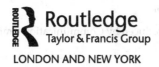

Routledge
Taylor & Francis Group

LONDON AND NEW YORK

First published 2016 by Karnac Books Ltd.

Published 2019 by Routledge
2 Park Square, Milton Park, Abingdon, Oxon OX14 4RN
52 Vanderbilt Avenue, New York, NY 10017, USA

Routledge is an imprint of the Taylor & Francis Group, an informa business

British Library Cataloguing in Publication Data

A C.I.P. for this book is available from the British Library

ISBN: 9781782203292 (pbk)

Edited, designed, and produced by Communication Crafts

CONTENTS

Margot Waddell & Jocelyn Catty

Since it was founded in 1920, the Tavistock Clinic has developed a wide range of developmental approaches to mental health which have been strongly influenced by the ideas of psychoanalysis. It has also adopted systemic family therapy as a theoretical model and a clinical approach to family problems. The Clinic is now the largest training institution in Britain for mental health, providing postgraduate and qualifying courses in social work, psychology, psychiatry, and child, adolescent, and adult psychotherapy, as well as in nursing and primary care. It trains about 1,700 students each year in over 60 courses.

The Clinic's philosophy aims at promoting therapeutic methods in mental health. Its work is based on the clinical expertise that is also the basis of its consultancy and research activities. The aim of this Series is to make available to the reading public the clinical, theoretical, and research work that is most influential at the Tavistock Clinic. The Series sets out new approaches in the understanding and treatment of psychological disturbance in children, adolescents, and adults, both as individuals and in families.

In *Making Room for Madness in Mental Health*, Marcus Evans has brought vividly to life one of the most challenging areas of clinical practice—namely, work with "madness", in its many forms. Drawing on decades of experience of direct clinical work, supervision, and consultation, he asks, tellingly, what happened to the "illness" when mental disorders became sanitized by the term "mental health". He painstakingly unpicks the layers of defences (in both patients and staff) that obscure the "madness" or psychosis in a range of disorders: psychotic disorders, eating disorders, personality disorders, self-harm, and hysteria. This is an unusual book in bringing together not just a range of clinical presentations but also complementary insights: those garnered through a career first in mental health nursing and then in psychoanalytic psychotherapy, and those arising from clinical psychotherapy and psychoanalytic consultation and supervision.

Marcus Evans makes a strong case for the importance of psychoanalytic supervision in mental health practice and its role in helping frontline staff to "tune in" to their patients' unconscious communications or the "psychotic wavelength". In so doing, he also makes the case for recognizing and confronting madness, and resisting the urge of so many mental health services to push madness out of sight as they try to persuade the patient to listen to reason. Striking vignettes enliven his arguments and show not only patients but also staff both in action and in thought (and sometimes in torment). In the chapters reflecting his own psychotherapeutic work, he shows as much insight and transparency about his own practice as he does, in other chapters, about the role of the supervision group for staff bringing their most challenging cases.

This book represents the insights and the lively thinking that result both from a rich career in "mental health" and psychoanalytic psychotherapy, and from clinical learning from the distinguished psychotherapists whom he acknowledges at the start of the book. Their insights permeate the book just as Marcus Evans's thoughtful attention must have permeated the supervision groups he describes. One of the teachers to whom he expresses particular gratitude is Mrs Edna O'Shaughnessy, and we are delighted that she agreed to write the Foreword to this powerful, inspiring, and ultimately compassionate book.

ACKNOWLEDGEMENTS

I qualified as a registered mental nurse in 1983, having completed my training at Springfield Hospital in South London. This training provided me with a professional ethic and basic knowledge of the medical model, and while this model provided a way of thinking about the broad categories of mental illness, it did not really offer me any way of understanding some of the patients' bizarre symptoms and behaviours. I was introduced to psychoanalysis by a psychotherapist at Springfield Hospital who worked on the wards. He suggested I read Melanie Klein's work, which opened my eyes to the idea that we all had an internal world that affects the way we think and relate. Since that time, my preoccupation has been the application of psychoanalytic thinking in mental health settings. I was fortunate to find a series of supervisors, colleagues, and mentors who supported my development from keen enthusiast to qualified practitioner. While I was a ward manager at St Giles Day Hospital, I was supervised on my first psychotherapy case by Dave Somekh, who has remained a mentor and friend to this day. In the mid-1980s, Duncan Maclean and Nick Temple encouraged my application to a course, "Seminars in Psychotherapy", run by John Steiner at the Tavistock Clinic. I also began analysis with Edith Hargreaves, who, over the many years

of my analysis, helped me to develop personally and professionally; I owe her a large debt of thanks. I subsequently worked in
the Maudsley Psychotherapy Unit while training at the Tavistock
Clinic as an adult psychoanalytic psychotherapist. I was fortunate
to be supervised by Sandy Bourne, Mani Lewis, Steve Dreyer,
Susan Davison, and Michael Feldman, and I qualified in 1996. Since
qualification, I have been privileged to be supervised by Leslie
Sohn, Richard Lucas, and John Steiner. I am proud to have been
one of the clinicians who treated patients as part of the Tavistock
Adult Depression Study. The clinical side of the study was run
by David Taylor, who provided a setting in which we could think
about and treat some of the most deprived and neglected patients
in the mental health system. I am also a member of the Fitzjohns
Unit in the Tavistock Adult Department, directed by David Bell and
managed by Birgit Kleeberg. This service provides twice-weekly
psychotherapy for patients who are not usually seen in outpatient
psychotherapy departments. Patients are often jointly managed
with local psychiatric services, and regular liaison with psychiatric services is essential to the success of the treatment. Edna
O'Shaughnessy runs a weekly clinical seminar, which supports the
work of the unit.

As Head of Nursing in the Tavistock and Portman NHS Foundation Trust and member of the Adult Department and, more
recently, as Associate Clinical Director of the Adolescent and Adult
departments, I have been working with and am supported by an
excellent group of colleagues and staff. I have also learnt from
the patients I have treated and the students I have taught and
supervised. This book has been a team effort going back over
many years, and I would like to thank Humphrey Mathews for
his perseverance during my nine attempts at English O-level, and
the Blackheath Rugby Cricket team, whose members have been
like a second family to me. I would also like to thank John Steiner,
Marilyn Lawrence, Professor Tom Burns, David Bell, Rob Harland,
Jenny Searle, Billie Joseph, Birgit Kleeberg, Maxine Dennis, Tom
Pennybacker, Nicky Kern, Carine Minne, Jo Stubley, Francesca
Hume, Anthony Garelick, Sally Davies, Michael Mercer, Philip
Stokoe, Paula Evans, Gerard Drennan, and, especially, Rinku Alam,
for reading the papers and giving helpful feedback from a psychi-
atric point of view. Louise Fruen has spared no effort in helping me

put these papers together and turn the phantasy into reality. Lucy Ettinger, my personal assistant at the Tavistock, found a few hours in my timetable to do some writing. Jocelyn Catty has worked tirelessly, reading draft after draft and providing long and detailed feedback. I also owe a huge debt of gratitude to my parents and all my family for their encouragement and support over the years and, last but by no means least, to my wife Sue, for her unswerving encouragement, spending countless hours doing endless edits and discussing issues raised. Sue has an invaluable and sometimes irritating quality of actually "thinking" and examining the facts rather than accepting ideas on the basis of fashion or reputation.

Chapters 2–6 are derived in part from articles previously published in *Psychoanalytic Psychotherapy*, copyright © The Association for Psychoanalytic Psychotherapy in the NHS, and are reprinted by permission of Taylor & Francis Ltd, www.tandfonline.com on behalf of The Association for Psychoanalytic Psychotherapy in the NHS:

Chapter 2: First published as: "Making Room for Madness in Mental Health: The Importance of Analytically Informed Supervision of Nurses and Other Mental Health Professionals" (Vol. 20, No. 1, 2006, pp. 16–29).

Chapter 3: First published as: "Being Driven Mad: Towards Understanding Borderline and Other Disturbed States of Mind Through the Use of the Counter-Transference" (Vol. 21, No. 3, 2007, pp. 216–232). [www.tandfonline.com/doi/full/10.1080/02668730701535578]

Chapter 4: First published as: "Pinned Against the Ropes: Understanding Anti-Social Personality-Disordered Patients Through Use of the Counter-Transference" (Vol. 25, No. 2, 2011, pp. 143–156).

Chapter 5: First published as: "Tuning into the Psychotic Wavelength: Psychoanalytic Supervision for Mental Health Professionals" (Vol. 22, No. 4, 2008, pp. 248–261).

Chapter 6: First published as: "The Role of Psychoanalytic Assessment in the Management and Care of a Psychotic Patient" (Vol. 25, No. 1, 2011, pp. 28–37).

ABOUT THE AUTHOR

Marcus Evans is a Consultant Adult Psychotherapist at the Tavistock and Portman NHS Foundation Trust, with thirty-five years' experience in mental health as a practitioner, lecturer, and manager. He qualified as a psychiatric nurse in 1983 and went on to occupy nursing posts as Charge Nurse of St Giles Day Hospital, Clinical Nurse Specialist in liaison psychiatry and para-suicide in Kings' College Hospital A&E, and Clinical Nurse Specialist in psychotherapy at the Bethlem and Maudsley hospitals. After qualifying as a psychotherapist at the Tavistock and Portman NHS Trust, he took up a post as Head of Nursing with a brief to develop the discipline within the Trust. He held the posts of Head of Nursing and Consultant Adult Psychotherapist until taking on the post of Associate Clinical Director of the Adult and Adolescent departments between 2011 and 2015. He has supervised, designed, developed, and taught outreach courses for frontline mental health staff in various settings for the last twenty-five years in many mental health trusts, including Camden and Islington and the Bethlem and Maudsley, and in Broadmoor. He was also one of the founding members of the Fitzjohn's Unit in the Adult Department at the Tavistock for the treatment of patients with severe and enduring mental health conditions and/or personality disorders; since stepping down as the Associate Clinical Director he has started working as a Consultant Adult Psychotherapist in the Portman Clinic. His passion is the application of psychoanalytic ideas to the treatment and care of patients in mental health settings.

PREFACE

I have been privileged to pursue my interest in the application of psychoanalytic ideas in mental health settings, first working as a clinical nurse specialist at the Bethlem and Maudsley Hospital and then as Head of Nursing at the Tavistock and Portman NHS Foundation Trust. These roles have allowed me to move between individual and group psychotherapeutic work and supervision of staff in mental health settings. I believe that it is important for frontline staff to be taught by practitioners who can speak from experience about the difficulties and dilemmas involved in the work, so my practice of on-going clinical work provides a regular reminder of the challenges involved. In my experience, mental health care always appears easier when practised at some distance from the frontline or in hindsight. Indeed, the danger is that the further you get from the action, the easier it becomes.

In this book I argue that, in addition to providing a helpful treatment for patients who suffer from serious psychological difficulties, the psychoanalytic model can help mental health staff develop a better understanding of their patients. Indeed, it can complement other models for thinking about patients and their disturbance. The psychoanalytic framework, which puts the transference–countertransference relationship at the centre of clinical practice, offers an important model for understanding staff–patient relationships and organizational dynamics. Mental health professionals need to be receptive to their patients' projections and communications, but these powerful projections can become overwhelming, especially for the nursing staff, who are often with their patients for long periods. The psychoanalytic model can also give mental health professionals a language for describing their experiences of, and interaction with, their patients. The model is developmental and provides a dynamic picture of the way different parts of the patient's self wrestle for control of the patient's mind over time. I believe this framework for understanding can help in the day-to-day management of these changes and fluctuations.

While I am primarily arguing for the relevance of psychoanalytic thinking in mental health settings, I also think it is important to stress the importance of psychiatry and psychiatric practice in supporting psychoanalytic work with patients in disturbed states of mind. Disturbed patients often need containment and active physical treatment in addition to understanding and thought.

I argue here that the categorization of mental illnesses into diagnoses provides a helpful clinical structure for thinking about them. I also believe that patients in disturbed states of mind sometimes need the containment of inpatient settings. Active treatments like medication or electroconvulsive therapy can help in ameliorating very disturbed mental states. Psychological treatments that attempt to actively intervene in the structure of the patient's mind and thinking also have an important part to play in the provision of good mental health systems, as do occupational therapy and rehabilitation, which are crucial in helping patients recover from breakdown. However, I would argue that the diagnosis and active interventions employed by psychiatry need to be accompanied by a receptive approach to treatment and care. Mental health professionals have to be interested in the meaning of their patients' symptoms and their verbal and physical communications, which may convey important information about patients' internal worlds and underlying conflicts. This receptive approach requires mental health professionals to make a switch from the active state of mind demanded by active interventions to the receptive state of mind required by the need to take in the patient's emotional state and underlying personality structure.

Following the Introduction to the book, which gives an overview of madness, mental health, and the mental health system,
I go on, in chapter 1, to use clinical examples to illustrate basic
psychoanalytic concepts that are referred to in subsequent chapters. Chapter 2 develops this theme by demonstrating the value
of psychoanalytic supervision for mental health professionals in
various community and inpatient settings.

In the following three chapters I focus on the more specific
clinical challenges posed by various patient groups. Chapter 3 is
concerned with the difficulties of working with patients in borderline states of mind, underlining the problems that staff may have
dealing with the concrete and powerful nature of their patients'
communications and actions. Chapter 4 examines the way patients
with antisocial personality disorder can act out their disturbances
in concrete ways designed to discharge psychic conflict and pain.
Chapter 5 describes working with patients who have a psychotic
illness and the way their often concrete communications can
crush any symbolic meaning. The discussion in all three chapters
includes illustrations of the transference and countertransference
issues involved in the care of these patient groups.

I then turn to clinical challenges encountered in the individual
psychotherapeutic treatment of patients with a severe or enduring
mental illness and/or personality disorder. Chapters 6, 7, and 8
use extracts from therapy to illustrate issues concerned with the
dynamics underlying the clinical presentation, focusing on the
relationship between patients' psychopathology, their patterns of
behaviour, and their ways of communicating; they also examine
problems encountered in the countertransference of the therapist.
Chapter 6 describes the assessment of a man with a serious psychotic condition. The assessment allowed me to develop an understanding of the patient's personality structure and risk profile. This
was then used in the establishment of a long-term treatment plan.
Chapter 7 describes the treatment of a patient who was involved
in compulsive, addictive, and life-threatening self-harming behaviour and my struggle to maintain a therapeutic stance in the face
of this extreme self-harming. Chapter 8 examines the treatment of
a severely ill anorexic woman whose fragmented means of communication posed a particular clinical problem in the treatment,
whereby as her therapist I felt pulled into a position where I

would want to rescue her from the deadly grip of her omnipotent defences.

Turning again to clinical work brought for psychoanalytic supervision, in Chapter 9 I describe the treatment of several patients who employed erotized defences against underlying depression and psychic pain. These patients often develop seductive relationships with mental health professionals, and the unconscious phantasies underlying these relationships are related to ideas about rescue and seduction. All of these clinical examples highlight the importance of tuning into the psychotic as well as the non-psychotic level of communication.

The clinical material presented is drawn from a combination of individual work and clinical supervisions undertaken in the NHS in the course of the past two decades. In the interest of confidentiality, examples are heavily disguised and come from an amalgam of different cases that exemplify specific clinical characteristics. The material from the supervision groups comes from various mental health trusts in which I have worked. Groups have been attended by a mixture of professionals, including nurses, psychologists, psychiatrists, housing officers, social workers, occupational therapists, mental health workers, and volunteers.

Finally, the Conclusion describes the value of psychoanalytic supervision for frontline professionals and for the treatment of patients with severe and enduring mental illness and/or personality disorders. It argues that individual psychoanalytic work complements supervision of frontline mental health professionals, and vice versa.

At the time of writing, there is enormous pressure on many mental health services to assess, treat, and discharge patients as speedily as possible—a pressure that can seriously interfere with the therapeutic relationship and the capacity of staff and patients to fully engage in their work together. While I observe and comment on the effects and risks of the current system, I have been consistently impressed and moved by the resilience, commitment, and interest in their work shown by staff in spite of this lack of resources and support.

Working with mental illness can be rewarding and enlightening. However, it is also disturbing, frightening, boring, frustrating, anxiety-provoking, and stupefying. We need to provide space for mental health professionals to reflect upon and think about their experiences on a day-to-day basis and to train clinicians to senior levels so that they can offer clinical supervision to frontline staff, to help them develop ideas about the meaning of their patients' symptoms and behaviours. Psychoanalysis offers a model for thinking about, and providing meaning for, the anxieties that drive us "out of our minds", and this can reduce the risk of thoughtless action. To some extent, this involves putting the madness back into mental health.

FOREWORD

Edna O'Shaughnessy

The title of this book, *Making Room for Madness in Mental Health: The Psychoanalytic Understanding of Psychotic Communication*, reveals at once the approach of its author, Marcus Evans, to treatment and to the psychoanalytic understanding of, and the nature of, the illness that he is concerned with—madness.

In a short paper, "On the Fear of Insanity", Roger Money-Kyrle called attention to the significant fact that "Most people fear contact with the insane" (1969, p. 434). This is the underlying reason, he thinks, why there has always been a tendency, among both ordinary people and professionals who work in the field of mental health, to keep insanity out of view. Money-Kyrle describes the terror and agony of madness and how the insane patient, too, cannot bear much contact with his state, a state whose transformations are mostly in the zones of hatred and destruction. Instead of contact with himself and others, the patient tries to defend himself with arrogance in an attempt to give himself strength and protection from danger and distress, and the humiliation of inferiority—this last being an especially painful and intolerable emotion. When he is in contact with others, he aims to dominate them, to have his delusions believed, and to attack and demolish their sanity. The patient is ill. So we say in common parlance: the balance of his

xxi

mind is disturbed—it has been taken over by death instincts. Our fears and concerns about the ill patient are compounded, Money-Kyrle suggests, because there is a mad part in all of us that could be recruited to join in with the patient's madness.

What has become, then, of the patient's life instincts in all their various constructive manifestations? The patient feels perhaps that they are somewhere out in space, or lodged inside other people, but broken and fragmented, changed, become hostile, as Bion (1957) described in "Differentiation of the Psychotic from the Non-Psychotic Personalities". We need to remember, too, as Melanie Klein said in "Notes on Some Schizoid Mechanisms" (1946), that while the patient has a vital need of schizoid mechanisms in order to be out of touch, to protect his ego and his self, yet, even so, at the same time, there almost always remains in the patient some wish and need to know, and also to be known and truthfully be understood.

All of this makes encounters with psychotic or borderline patients complex and uncertain, at times even dangerous, both for the patient and for those who are around him. Marcus Evans has written this book from his long practical experience of working with patients alongside psychoanalytic and other therapeutic colleagues in psychiatric settings. He begins with an excellent overview, in which he sets out his general position. One of his chief contentions is that many patients are open to, and can benefit from, a psychoanalytic understanding of their psychic situation, but that there are also likely to be times when the patient, and sometimes the therapist too, may need the help of other approaches, including medication, to "keep the insanity out of view" and so bring much-needed relief, possibly from risk of suicide or violence. Thus psychotherapy and psychiatry, Marcus Evans believes, are dependent on one another in the treatment of patients with the severe personality disorders of mental illness.

Furthermore, while many ill patients can benefit from psychotherapy, all patients, he contends, are in need of mental health staff who are able to be interested in the emotional aspects of minds, their own and those of others, and who can tune in to a psychotic level of communication. Marcus Evans shows how much staff need to be able to carry: projections from patients of unwanted aspects of themselves, provocative behaviour, psychic pressures to enact, in reality, bizarre phantasies and hostile divisive attacks on the staff.

In his clinical illustrations it emerges how essential it is to support staff by providing supervision and discussion, so that through an understanding of what is happening, they may become able to resist the temptation to act out with patients or with one another. All of this brings into view an important and particular conception of workers in mental health organizations as all, of necessity— if to different degrees—being involved with patients. While this requires a willingness to accept psychological burdens, there is a notable gain as it adds much to the interest and status of the work.

A series of vivid clinical illustrations of patients, each with a particular type of disturbance, forms the main part of the book. Marcus Evans shows how the powerful insane forces driving the patient impact on the therapist. Often, in these narratives, it is the author himself at work, but he also describes various characteristic situations involving other mental health workers. He shows how by not *doing* something, by paying attention, listening, trying to understand the unconscious communications—perhaps (say) the nature of the huge anxiety in a desperate, bizarre presentation—we may reach the patient, who may then be able to make of it a healing experience of being understood.

This is a book of great value for all concerned, in whatever way, with the treatment of severely mentally ill patients. We see the problems and sufferings of the patients, their strange and disturbing engagements with staff, and the resulting problems and need for support of the staff. But the paramount fact, as Marcus Evans shows, is the way that the psychoanalytic method does not keep insanity out of view, but tries to offer madness a habitat and human understanding.

Introduction

Madness is the colloquial and sometimes derogatory term used to describe insanity: the fragmented and chaotic state of mind of the person who becomes detached from the consensual view of reality. In the first instance, the mental health care system has to provide a setting where madness and anxieties about madness can be managed safely by empathic and thoughtful staff. In many ways this is a natural process that takes place in the encounter between patient and mental health professional. However, in this book I argue that good mental health care—and treatment—needs to go beyond this important first step, by trying to understand the relationship between patients' presentations and their personalities. Indeed, highly disturbed patients need to be cared for by mental health professionals who are interested in and committed to understanding the meaning behind the presenting problem. Recovery will depend upon patients' ability to reclaim their capacity for psychological thought and insight.

The development of insight can, however, be a persecutory process in itself, as patients become aware of the fragmentation of their minds and their detachment from shared reality. Post-traumatic depression is a common symptom in patients in the process of recovering from a serious and enduring mental ill-ness, as they often feel they are unable to face the full extent of their psychological difficulties. They may also worry that they are unlovable, untreatable, unbearable, or damaging to others, and they may, out of desperation, seek ideal or magical solutions to their problems—solutions that may, in turn, impede the recovery process as patients develop a psychic structure designed to avoid painful realities. John Steiner (1993a) makes the point that these defensive organizations need to be respected and understood, as they provide respite from demanding anxieties that have to do with fragmentation on the one hand and depression on the other. Con-sequently, insight into the nature of patients' difficulties often has to be developed and contained by the mental health professional in the first instance. The demanding and difficult task of reflecting on such communications needs to be central to the mental health professional's clinical work in order to help develop ideas about underlying conflicts and difficulties. Understanding the patient's use of defences helps professionals to make sense of what might have been disregarded as inexplicable behaviour. The risk is that patients' communications are dismissed as secondary to an illness and thus "un-understandable" (Jaspers, 1913) rather than inher-ently meaningful and an opportunity to learn about the patients and enable patients to learn more about themselves.

Although in many ways empathic understanding is a natural process, understanding underlying conflicts requires space to take a step back and reflect. Professionals need time for clinical discus-sion and supervision in order to support the development of ideas about the underlying nature of a patient's disturbance. This activity needs, in turn, to be supported by clinical and managerial struc-tures in order to help staff contain the inevitable anxieties inherent in their work. Psychoanalytically informed supervision and train-ing provides a model for thinking about conscious and uncon-scious communications as they are expressed in the clinical setting. Through its understanding of transference and countertransference phenomena, it also puts the therapeutic relationship at the centre of the work. Using examples from supervision groups and indi-vidual patients in psychotherapy, I illustrate how a psychoanalytic approach to mental health can complement other ways of thinking about practice and management. I show how this understanding helps to develop and maintain therapeutic factors, while reducing the risk of poor clinical management decisions, which are often due to a more cursory understanding of the clinical need. The psychoanalytic model also provides a way of considering psychotic communications and levels of thinking in the patient's personality.

Traditionally, mental illness has been divided into neurotic and psychotic disorders. According to Freud,

> one of the features which differentiates a neurosis from a psychosis is the fact that in a neurosis the ego, in its dependency on reality, suppresses a piece of the id (of instinctual life), whereas in psychosis, this same ego, in the service of the id, withdraws from a piece of reality. [Freud, 1924e, p. 183]

O'Shaughnessy (1992, p. 89) puts this succinctly: "in neurosis, the relation to reality is retained at the cost of instinctual repression, while in psychosis the relation to reality is lost". She goes on to say that "Freud also became convinced of a proclivity for psychosis in all of us."

In this book, I argue that psychotic thinking and structures lie beneath most severe neurotic conditions, and clinicians need to try to tune in to the psychotic as well as the neurotic wavelength (Lucas, 2009e).

The ego, a psychic structure made up of internalized relationships, comes into existence at the very beginning of life. The ego may be more or less robust, depending on how these relationships are internalized, and this is determined by both constitutional and environmental factors. The term "breakdown" is used to describe the traumatic loss of an important internal structure (the ego), which either leaves the individual feeling overwhelmed by psychotic anxieties about fragmentation or leads to psychological collapse in the ego's functioning—a collapse that may have been precipitated by a traumatic loss in the individual's external world as it reverberates in the internal world.

From a psychoanalytic perspective, psychotic anxiety resulting from the loss threatens to overwhelm the individual's ego, and there is a collapse in the ego's capacity to manage the relationship between internal and external reality. In an attempt to regain control of this chaotic situation, some individuals may take drastic physical and/or psychological action: patients may, for example, act out violently in order to expel the overwhelming internal state, thereby forcing others to take control of their lives. Other individuals might develop an apparently neurotic mental structure that is, in fact, a rigid defensive organization designed to keep out any contact with reality, including the possibility of genuine relationships with others, which are experienced as too threatening. The debilitating nature of this neurotic defence interferes with individuals' capacity to function in an ordinary way, again forcing others to take responsibility. Alternatively, depressed individuals may collapse into a state of self-blame and hopeless infantile dependence or of catatonic withdrawal. Patients whose minds fragment into psychotic states develop delusional systems in an attempt to gather the mind together and provide coherence and continuity. The delusional system binds the fragmented parts of the mind together into a "coherent" belief system created by the patient—a belief system that is, however, based on a psychic structure that bears no obvious relation to external reality.

Patients' breakdown

Patients are admitted into the mental health system when the nature of their breakdown means that they can no longer be contained in their usual setting. They need a safe place where the effects of their chaotic mental states and unpredictable behaviours can be managed safely. The Greek word "asylum", meaning "place of safety", was used to describe Victorian psychiatric hospitals that housed large numbers of patients until the 1980s. The solid asylum walls were designed to provide a concrete container for the patients' fragmented minds while keeping them safe from harm. Steiner emphasized the strengths and weaknesses of "the brick mother"—the term Henry Rey used to describe the Maudsley Hospital—in that the solid walls provided stability but could also be hard, cold, and unyielding (Steiner & Harland, 2011, p. 16). Steiner argued that the walls of the asylum needed to be softened through a human approach based on understanding.

The asylum also represented the place where all the mad elements of society could be projected—the "bin" where madness could be discarded. In the 1960s, Goffman, a sociologist, described in his book, *Asylums*, the way asylums institutionalized patients into a chronic state of dependence upon an inhumane system (Goffman, 1968). He argued that patients needed to be deinstitutionalized. In the 1970s, psychiatry was led to believe that new drugs would cure mental illness and there would be little need for long-term psychiatric beds. In the 1980s, this new optimism regarding the treatment of long-term mental illness, together with developments in social psychiatry, led to the closure of the asylums, and care for the severe and enduringly mentally ill moved from institutions to community settings. While some of the changes that have taken place over the past three to four decades have been helpful, in my view a fundamental clinical problem remains. Hinshelwood emphasized psychotic patients' assault on meaning and meaningful communication, withdrawing instead into a delusional world of their own creation. Bell and Novakovic (2013) comment that "Meaninglessness is like a vacuum, and nature abhors it—or, rather, human nature does" (2013, p. 197).

Hinshelwood (2013) describes the difficulty mental health professionals and families experience, having to bear the impact of psychotic communication. Deprived of ordinary meaningful contact, mental health professionals can withdraw into rather mechanistic and detached ways of thinking and relating to their patients. Patients with chronic psychotic conditions and the accompanying negative symptoms need help to resist the regressive pull away from the persecutory demands of reality into a delusional world of their own creation. This regressive tendency needs to be worked with by mental health professionals who understand that patients have to be helped to face the demands of reality in a sympathetic, sensitive, but persistent way. Mental health professionals need to engage their patients in this struggle over time. The families who care for people who suffer from long-term psychotic states also need help and support in managing this long-term condition. This is why regular occupational therapy, organized activities, and visits from community psychiatric nurses (CPNs), delivered either on inpatient units or in community settings such as day hospitals or recovery centres, form an essential part of patients' recovery.

The shift from institutional to community care

Relationships with community mental health professionals and clinical teams have, to some extent, replaced the asylum, and yet community care has never been adequately resourced. In an article for the Centre for Health and the Public Interest, Bell points out that the closure of psychiatric beds has resulted in huge pressure on psychiatric inpatient wards. In the United Kingdom there is currently 100% occupancy on many wards, with 80% of the patients held under mental health legislation (Bell, 2013). Many inpatient units have very little occupational therapy available, and high levels of drug abuse and violence in some areas can create environments dominated by custodial rather than therapeutic principles. One ward manager from an inpatient psychiatric ward told a work discussion group that there had been 18 incidents of violence on her ward during the course of one week, including one occasion when the staff team was held hostage by a patient wielding an axe.

With inpatient units often completely filled with those who are acutely ill, the shortage of beds creates pressure to discharge even patients with serious and enduring mental illnesses back to primary care at the earliest possible opportunity, resulting in a situation where some patients do not have any time to consolidate their improvement, and their early discharge puts pressure on community psychiatric teams to manage high levels of disturbance. Caseloads in community settings have increased as a result of reductions in funding, and many services are under pressure. In community mental health settings, staff are often exposed to patients' anxiety, pain, and disturbance without the supportive, if rather rigid, container formerly provided by traditional institutional settings. There are conflicting pressures within the system, which impinge on the professional's clinical judgement or capacity to think objectively. On the one hand, mental health professionals are expected to keep patients out of hospital, and admission is often looked upon as a failure; on the other, community staff are expected to provide assurances about patient risk management in the community.

Anxiety about the extent of their damaged minds, both internally in phantasy and externally in reality, can overwhelm patients with despair, driving them to resort to manic defences based on magical thinking in order to deny underlying feelings of guilt or impotence. Psychotic elements of the mind can promote unrealistic, omnipotent ideas of cure and self-sufficiency, while parts of the self that acknowledge the need for healthy dependency are attacked and undermined. Patients in manic states often believe that they can deal with their underlying anxieties about damage by magical means. This includes putting psychic or physical distance between themselves and the problem, as if difficulties could be located in a geographical area and then left behind. In practical terms, this can lead to absconding, or planning an unrealistic journey, or a change of job or partner. The problem with these mechanisms is that eventually, when the defence can no longer be maintained, they break down.

Patients who become aware of the extent of their difficulties, in addition to feelings of anxiety, loss, and despair, are also prone to feelings of humiliation. Indeed, the dependence upon professionals and the inevitable imbalance in authority can highlight patients' feelings of inferiority. The fact that mental health professionals are required to assess patients' state of mind and functioning can also exacerbate feelings of being looked down on, judged, and/or shamed. Professionals need to be sensitive to these feelings and, whenever possible, help support patients in managing them. If professionals act in ways that are insensitive to patients' shame and humiliation, this may exacerbate historical feelings of resentment and unfairness in relation to authority. If these issues are not understood, they can become the locus of a grievance between patient and professional; this undermines the therapeutic relationship, which is central to the process of recovery. However, even if professionals are sensitive to these issues, the imbalance of power in the relationship can still inflame these dynamics; this becomes most evident when professionals are required to execute their professional role and responsibility.

In order to avoid the dynamics outlined above, professionals may find themselves adopting approaches that are affected by unconscious forces, as they attempt to avoid any stance that differentiates them from the patient. This loss of differentiation and reluctance to take up a position of professional authority can lead to an erosion of professional practice. An example of this can be seen when mental health clinicians reassure patients that their thinking is quite normal or "nothing to worry about", even when patients say they are becoming unwell. This reassurance leaves responsibility for the problem with the part of the patient that is in touch with the extent of the difficulty. Numerous serious untoward incident investigations highlight service failures to listen to patients who had reported that they were feeling unwell and in danger of harming themselves and/or others. Investigations also point to the fact that relatives are often ignored when they recognize signs of breakdown in the patient. Issues surrounding the patient's right to confidentiality can interfere with information gathering, even though good practice demands that a full assessment of someone with a serious and enduring mental illness should include an interview with relatives who know the patient. A psychodynamic understanding can help us to see the powerful unconscious dynamics that may lead to certain information being passed over in favour of collusion to ignore serious illness. Exploring the powerful emotions at play within treating teams is often a helpful and realistic way of understanding mistakes rather than a response that seeks to attribute blame.

The role of diagnosis

There are mixed views on the importance of diagnosis within the mental health profession: some parts of the system use diagnostic criteria as an organizing principle that guides treatment and approach, whereas other parts of the system are moving away from what is seen as the paternalism of the medical model. For example, nurses from several different mental health trusts have said that newly qualified nurses get very little training in diagnosis or the medical model. The rationale for this change in practice seems to be related to the belief that diagnosis can be stigmatizing.

Patients also have mixed views on diagnosis, with some disliking the idea because they believe that it will be used to label them and discount their views, while others demand a diagnosis that will explain their condition. It is certainly true that thinking about the diagnosis can be used to distance the professional from the patient and contribute to a rather mechanistic approach. It is also true that a rigid interpretation of the medical model can discourage thinking about the person behind the illness. However, the medical model does help professionals to categorize and organize groups of signs and symptoms into diagnostic categories with different treatment requirements and prognosis. Unwittingly, professionals may be tempted to collude with these ideas in order to avoid painful realities about patients' clinical condition. While mental health professionals need to be sensitive to patients' feelings of humiliation and despair, this collusion can leave patients on their own with their anxieties about the extent of their difficulties. It also gives the impression that the profession cannot bear the anxiety and despair involved in facing mental illness. Indeed, I sometimes find myself wondering where we thought the "illness" had gone when we changed from the term "mental illness" to "mental health". Although the change in description did represent a helpful attempt to reduce stigma, it can become aligned with a wish to get rid of the idea that the patient suffers from a serious psychological difficulty.

Minne (2003) outlined the way both staff and patients in forensic settings often push patients' violent or risky behaviour out of mind. This can then lead to a dangerous situation, as awareness of the risk, which has been pushed "out of mind", may suddenly return in the form of violent acting out. Certainly, if you read government policy documents for mental health, there is very little mention of mental illness or psychosis—a state of ignorance and denial that leaves professionals, patients, and society at risk, as we are in danger of forgetting what we are dealing with. The painful fact is that mental illness is, by its very nature, unpredictable: the only reliable indicator of future risk is knowledge of patients' history, including their past risk behaviour and their current mental state—in other words, knowing patients in as great a depth as possible.

An important part of any patient's recovery is based on the capacity to mourn the loss of the ideal self and to face painful realities. This involves taking back aspects of the self that have been denied, split off, and projected. There are inevitably cycles in this recovery as it moves between periods of development and mental integration and periods of disintegration and regression—a process that is precarious and may lead to feelings of guilt and despair, followed by fragmentation and/or a retreat into paranoia, which acts as a defence against depressive feelings about the damage done. Patients may also retreat into a defensive state of grievance as they feel that they are victims of their illness or of their abusive histories and consequently cannot and should not be held accountable. Steiner (1993a) has outlined the way patients develop psychic retreats designed to defend them from the demands of development and insight on the one hand, and fears of fragmentation on the other. Patients need periods when they are protected from the demands of integration; their defences need to be respected, and they need time to gather their resources before further progress can be made. The problem with this is that it takes time—a commodity that is increasingly squeezed by financial pressures and the idealistic demands of patients and staff alike.

Institutional defences

Jaques (1955) and Menzies (1960) pioneered work in applying psychoanalytic thinking to the study of organizations and social systems. Menzies' seminal paper, "The Functioning of Social Systems as a Defence against Anxiety", was based on consultation with the nursing hierarchy in a large teaching hospital. She looked at the relationship between the social system and anxieties inherent in the work. The nurses' work meant that they were in close proximity to patients who were either ill or dying, and they were confronted on a regular basis with their own anxieties about illness and death. Menzies described a social system that fragmented and distanced the relationship between nurses and the patient. Anxiety became detached from its source and attached to rituals and rigid practices within the organization. The institution developed an overly defensive organizational structure designed to avoid anxiety rather than think and feel. In mental health services, the main anxiety, which is largely denied, is concerned with the unpredictability of mental illness.

In a supervision group, a CPN described how ritualized and fragmented their assessment process had become, as various admission forms gathering information dominated the interview.

The forms included basic demographic information, a risk-assessment form, a smoking-cessation form, a form categorizing the patient's problem, and a research study into projected level of need. By the time these forms have been completed, there is no time to talk to the patient. Although we have dismantled the institutions, we seem to be constructing a new set of defences designed to keep patients, their disturbance, and their illness at a safe distance. A wall of paper has replaced the walls and jangling keys of the asylum. Many practitioners complain that they are driven to the use of defensive forms of practice to avoid being blamed if mistakes or oversights occur. In a paper on risk assessment, Lucas (2003) outlined the way in which staff anxieties about blame and fears of reprisals from administration can contribute towards burnout in the workforce. Consequently, practitioners can become emotionally unavailable and detached from their patients and themselves, falling into thoughtless patterns of behaviour that avoid the development of understanding or meaning. This type of defensive thinking and behaviour can reduce professionals' immediate anxieties about blame and painful contact with disturbed and disturbing patients; however, in the longer term, ritualized practice by the clinician leaves the patient feeling isolated, while the practitioner feels demoralized or detached.

Over recent years, funding for mental health services in the United Kingdom has been consistently cut more than that for acute medicine. This reduction in services can drive commissioners to push for reductions in staffing levels and grades of staff, closure of beds, and reduction in treatment lengths. The shortage of resources can encourage the employment of manic defences in the mental health system. Treatment length is increasingly based on limited resources rather than on clinical evidence. Patients with serious and enduring mental health conditions alternate between various states of mind and need services that can support them in different ways over long periods of time. However, I would argue that, whatever the intervention, each patient's state should be seen and understood within the context of its overall development and history. Mental health professionals need to try to take a long-term view of their patients, including the fact that they may move in and out of illness over a period of time. Managers and commissioners need to be helped to understand that mental illness is damaging and serious and at times dangerous and unpredictable, and so usually it cannot be managed on a short-term, one-off basis. However, in the attempt to reduce costs, the squeeze on the time available for teaching, supervision, and/or case discussion undermines the time and structures necessary to support the reflective capacity of individuals and teams, thereby removing the structures that support clinicians' capacity to digest experience. There is a danger of creating, in their place, a system that increases the distance between patients and their suffering and the mental health professional.

Case example

A mental health volunteer presented the case of Mr A, who had a history of homelessness. He described the man as a lost soul, without personality or identity.

"I go round to see him every week. Mr A is completely isolated, rarely speaks, and spends his days staring at the wall. I think he is hearing or seeing things, as occasionally he responds to things going on his mind by muttering or laughing to himself. Mr A does not wash, and the flat is filthy. I have tried to get him assessed by various different services, because I think he is ill, but everyone says there is nothing wrong with him. When they ask him about psychotic symptoms, he denies them and says he has dreams in front of his eyes. On one occasion, out of desperation, I took a mental health professional around to Mr A's flat, so she would see the state of his home, but Mr A would not open the door. The professional said that Mr A did not have to let her in, as this was his choice, and the visit was abandoned."

We can see here how Mr A denied the nature of his psychotic illness by keeping it to himself. He normalized his hallucinations by calling them "dreams in front of my eyes". The negative effects of the schizophrenia led to him withdrawing from contact with the external world into a delusional world of his own creation. The patient's denial and rationalization of his illness, combined with the pressure on the mental health professional to restrict the numbers on the caseload, can lead to a collusion between the mental health services and the patient. Patients with serious and enduring mental illness need services and professionals who are able to listen, take in, and bear the pain of their psychological disturbance. However, the challenge for mental health professionals is to work out which part of the patient is talking, and with what aim. Is it the healthy part of the patient, which is in touch with psychic reality and the need for help, or the psychotic part, which employs denial and rationalization to justify its argument and conceal the real goal of manic self-sufficiency; or is it the perverse part, which wishes to interfere with the establishment of a truthful picture, or an infantile part that wishes to maintain a position of infantile dependence? Healthy aspects of the mind that contain awareness and insight can wrestle with psychotic elements of the mind in a dynamic struggle.

The distinction between illness and health is useful when determining whether the patient's disturbance has moved from something that convention would describe as "within the normal range" to something that would be deemed to be "abnormal". This helps psychiatrists to make decisions about the necessity for treatment and their degree of responsibility for the patient, and also whether the severity of the condition warrants compulsory detention in order to care for them. The dividing line between illness and health provides the clarity necessary for making decisions about appropriate action. However, this sort of medical categorization does not provide a model for thinking about the dynamic interplay between different parts of the personality operating within and influencing the patient's mind. In the example described above, the mental health professional listens to Mr A's denial and rationalization of his illness and decides that he is well enough to make his own decisions; this leaves the patient untreated and the volunteer with responsibility for a man who is out of touch with the level of his disturbance. Thus professional and patient alike avoid painful thinking about the patient and the patient's state of mind.

Manic defences in mental health

New treatment approaches are usually based on the germ of a good idea. However, I would argue that anxieties about the limitations of treatment, combined with anxieties about limited resources, are always threatening to ignite omnipotent defences within the mental health profession. Consequently, new approaches that require the allocation of stretched financial resources in order to be implemented are often accompanied by rather overblown claims in relation to therapeutic outcome and expectations—an "over-valuing" of the new that is usually accompanied by a subtle denigration of old methods. Mental health professionals are encouraged to believe that the latest philosophy is going to revolutionize the delivery of mental health treatment and care. Inevitably, there is a tendency to "throw the baby out with the bath water" as new ways of thinking can be adopted in a wholesale and rather unexamined way.

The current "recovery model", for instance, is based on the idea that mental health services and professionals need to support and enhance the patient's capacities, rather than allowing the patient to become passively dependent upon a system that focuses on an illness model. Emphasis is placed on the need for hope and belief in the process of change. In my experience, there is a great deal to be said for this approach, as focusing entirely on patients' psychopathology can make the clinical situation worse. Patients often need professionals to identify and support healthy aspects of their mind and personality. Indeed, even very unwell patients can feel better when they are able to join in with ordinary, meaningful activities, and this is an important part of the process of recovery.

The danger is that the recovery model can be used in a defensive way that denies painful clinical realities—namely, the fact that healthy aspects of a patient's mind and personality live in a dynamic relationship with other more destructive parts of the self. Many patients with a severe and enduring mental illness feel persecuted by their illness and wish to leave behind the services and treatments that remind them of their difficulties. Patients will sometimes persuade staff to discharge them from mental health services, as if they are cured, only to suffer a further breakdown, which necessitates readmission within a short period of time. This problem can be exacerbated by mental health professionals and services who believe that dependency is unhealthy, rather than being an essential part of all human relationships. Patients can, of course, develop malignant or unhealthy dependencies, but the capacity to depend upon others is an essential ingredient of mental health. Indeed, where the patient is able to form a healthy dependency on mental health professionals, it can herald the start of their recovery. *

The danger of concrete thinking in psychiatric settings

In the last two decades, there has been a conscious attempt to shift the emphasis from the professional towards the patient voice. There are many things to admire about this shift, and it should go without saying that mental health services need to tune in to the preoccupations of the patients they treat and care for. However, if patients' complaints and demands are dealt with in a concrete way, with little or no critical thought or examination, it can undermine the clinical container necessary for the treatment of patients in disturbed and disturbing states of mind.

Case example

With a mixture of frustration and distress, a ward manager from an acute admission ward talked in a supervision group about a situation that had occurred on her ward the previous month.

A patient had complained that he saw his primary nurse (a young female agency nurse) having sex with another male patient in the hospital grounds. The complaint was reported to the manager, who, in turn, reported the matter to the chief executive's office. The agency nurse was automatically suspended from further work within the trust, without any discussion of the case or preliminary examination of the facts. The nurse was not informed why she had been suspended, and other members of the staff team were forbidden from contacting her until the complaint had been resolved. The ward manager was upset because she already had problems staffing her ward, and she felt that this woman was a promising young nurse who had considered applying for a permanent post. Members of the staff team were interviewed, as well as the other patient concerned, until it was eventually established that the allegation was false.

The suspended nurse was, however, so traumatized by the events that she decided to leave the profession.

The patient was a man with a dual diagnosis and a long history of making sexually inappropriate passes at attractive female nurses. His mother had been a prostitute, who put him into care at an early age. Feeling let down by the agency nurse, who had only made a temporary commitment to the ward, the patient was jealous of her contact with other patients. The patient thus defended himself from anxiety about dependence and separation by sexualizing his contact with the nurse. As long as the patient felt that he was in control of the nurse's mind and central to her preoccupations, this situation was relatively stable. However, when he observed the nurse caring for other patients, he felt that he had lost his control over her, which exposed him to feelings of anxiety related to separateness and dependence. These anxieties resulted from deep-seated insecurities rooted in a personal history of being abandoned by his mother, and jealousy of his mother's relationships with other men, who paid for sex. In this state of mind, the patient had violently projected aspects of his internal world onto the external world, and, in the process, he lost the capacity to differentiate between internal and external reality. The violence of these projections meant that he lost the capacity to symbolize. The external object (the agency nurse) was felt to be the same as the internal object (the prostitute mother), rather than a symbolic representation.

This example shows how the therapeutic relationship with a difficult patient can haemorrhage into the political and managerial system in an unhelpful way, damaging patient care and staff morale. The institutional protocol, which demanded that the nurse must be suspended immediately as a result of the complaint, seriously undermined the nursing team's morale. This over-sensitive complaints tripwire also undermines the staff's belief that senior management trust them to know the difference between a legitimate complaint and psychosis or re-enactments of past traumas. By responding so concretely, the institution unwittingly re-enacts the patient's own history as the paternal aspects of management fail to protect and support the maternal aspects of nursing care for the patient. The institution's failure of symbolization also leaves the patient at risk of having to deal with guilt about his damaging accusation and the staff at risk of having their professional morale damaged.

The role of medication

Medication can play an essential role in reducing persecutory anxiety, which overwhelms the patient's capacity to think in an ordinary way. This reduction in the influence of disturbed states of mind in the acute phase of the illness may then enable patients to reclaim their capacity to think about themselves in relation to reality. This can be a great relief to patients who may be persecuted by the knowledge that they have lost their minds.

A reestablishment of patients' capacity to think about reality is the first stage of recovery; it paves the way for the second stage: coming to terms with the breakdown. This stage involves the painful psychological work of mourning, as patients have to come to terms with the fact that they have lost their minds. The first stage of recovery can take place in a matter of days, weeks, or months. Most people recover their capacity to think relatively quickly, whereas the second stage may take quite a bit longer, and some patients may never be able to come to terms with losing their mind and their sense of well-being. Medication can help with the pain involved in the second stage, as patients might understandably fear further breakdown as a result of the mourning process. Patients' recovery in both stages may be supported by good nursing care, occupational therapy, and psychotherapy, as well as relationships with significant others. Some patients, however, believe they are so damaged or fragile that they cannot bear the pain and anxiety involved in the second stage of recovery. Instead, they seek magical solutions that look to bypass the process of mourning. Many patients put pressure on the psychiatrist to provide a magic pill—medication that will cure them in isolation. When this fails to provide the ideal cure, patients often blame the type or dose of medication and ask for a change, still avoiding having to come to terms with their breakdown from a psychological perspective.

The wish to meet patients' demands for a cure, combined with the shortage of time and therapeutic resources, may also contribute to a tendency by mental health professionals to view the role of medication in isolation—as if medication could cure the condition on its own, without any other form of therapeutic work. In this way, the idealization of medication can be used to protect both clinician and patient from painful psychic realities. This over-valued belief in the role of medication is often reflected in the amount of time spent in clinical meetings discussing its influence in isolation, without reference to the significance of nursing care, occupational therapy, or participation in a patient's recovery programme.

There is no doubt that medication is central to the treatment of patients in acutely disturbed states of mind, and it also has an important role to play in the management of some chronic psychiatric conditions. However, medication does not address the underlying causes of mental illness, and patients need other forms of therapeutic work and support as part of their treatment. For example, the remission of "positive symptoms" in psychotic conditions as a result of medication is sometimes mistaken for cure. Mental health professionals can forget that the "negative symptoms" of psychotic states and patients' withdrawal from the external world are as important—if not more so—as the presence or absence of positive symptoms. The patient usually needs active rehabilitation and support from mental health professionals to enable a reengagement with external reality and life. Although medication may reduce intrusive symptoms and thus increase patients' availability for therapeutic engagement, it cannot replace the role of nurses and occupational therapists.

Lucas (2009a) described psychotic patients as needing an exoskeleton around them that would help pull them out of their withdrawn, negativistic state and into contact with external reality. Staff who work with chronic patients with serious and enduring illnesses need to be highly motivated and be prepared to engage with them through a process of rehabilitation over weeks, months, and sometimes years. I would argue that this painstaking therapeutic work is as important as the medication in helping patients to recover from their illness.

The therapeutic relationship

Continuity of care is a prerequisite for good mental health and treatment, because it allows clinicians and patients time to get to know one another. It gives clinicians time to gather together facts, impressions, and the experience of being with the patient and to deepen their understanding of the patient; it also gives patients an opportunity to bring different elements of them-selves over time. The "therapeutic relationship" between profes-sional and patient can provide an opportunity to bring back into mind what has been pushed out. This process may need to go on within the professional's mind in the first instance before patients can be expected to take back an awareness of their state. This involves a process of taking in patients' states of mind and pro-jections through observations and contact with their emotional and physical state (Fabricius, 1991). Using their own internal experience of suffering and anxieties about illness and damage, professionals form identifications with the patients. They convey understanding of the patients' anxiety and pain through a com-passionate and thoughtful attitude. When things are going well, this identification with patients is based on the patient being a symbolic representation of the clinician's own damaged objects. This confusion of the internal world with the external world can lead either to manic and/or to heroic attempts on the part of the professional to cure the patient or to a situation where profes-sionals feel defeated by the impossibility of the task. They may develop a hard external skin that gives the impression of cruel indifference as a way of keeping patients and their difficulties at a distance (Evans, 2014).

The capacity to move between empathic identification with the patients' suffering and objective professionalism is an essential pro-cess in maintaining a mature and healthy clinical approach. Sup-port to the clinician in this process needs to be provided through clinical discussion, reflective practice, and good management. On the one hand, these opportunities can help professionals to sepa-rate from the effect of their patients and restore an objective clinical approach; on the other, staff who have become hardened are helped to reflect more on the emotional impact of the clinical contact. Thus, professionals are supported in maintaining the difference between the patient as a helpful symbolic representation of the professional's own damaged figures and an unhelpful concrete equation.

A CPN told a supervision group about a patient in a violent psychotic state, who had recently been admitted to the locked ward for the fourth time in as many years.

> The patient had been discharged from hospital six months earlier. He felt stigmatized by his psychiatric label and didn't like the side-effects of his medication. Within five weeks he persuaded the CPN to discharge him from follow-up, and soon after this stopped taking his medication. Several months later, he was detained under mental health legislation and admitted to the locked psychiatric ward because of his violent behaviour. The nurse explained that she did not like to feel that her contact with the patient reminded him of his illness. The patient also felt that on-going contact with psychiatric services undermined his self-esteem and view of himself as better and as strong. Discharging the patient also provided a space on the CPN's overcrowded caseload.

> The origins of this particular breakdown started when the patient persuaded the CPN that he was well enough to stop having psychiatric follow-up and discontinued his medication. The psychosis had already started to re-establish its hold within the patient's personality, as evidenced by his wishes, which denied any knowledge of his history, illness, or dependence upon the services or the likely outcome of these actions.

Professionals obviously have to listen to patients and consider their views, but the latter can make unrealistic demands, based on a wish to deny painful realities. Rather than listening to these wishes and attempting to understand the patient's conflict and painful psychological state, the mental health system sometimes colludes by responding concretely. The capacity to depend upon others, which includes an awareness of limitations, is an important part of any patient's treatment, care, and potential for recovery. When patients reject the opportunity to form a helpful dependence, they may be forced back into the grip of more psychotic parts of their personality. This can increase the risk, and the danger of relapse as their underlying pathology goes unrecognized. Patients' wish to return to a self-sufficient state of mind that denies underlying difficulties in an attempt to get away from the reality of their dependence on psychiatric support and treatment is understandable, as dependence may leave them feeling small, damaged, or humiliated. However, discharge from services may leave patients in the hands of psychotic aspects of themselves without the support of psychiatric services.

Good clinical work depends upon professionals' capacity to listen to their patients while maintaining a space in which they are able consider their own point of view. In this space, the professional can reflect on the clinical facts and form an opinion based upon knowledge of each patient's personality, history, illness and diagnosis, patterns of behaviour, and relationships. It is also important that discussion takes place among the clinical team in order that the views of colleagues and their own clinical experience, thoughts, and feelings about the patient are brought together. I have found that the psychoanalytic approach can then help practitioners to make sense of this information. The challenge is to create structures and trainings that support professionals in this difficult and complex task.

Making room for mental illness in mental health

To some extent, the mental health professionals' capacity to think about their patients has replaced the asylum as the "container". The "therapeutic relationship" should be one of the main pillars of treatment. However, many mental health professionals receive very little training in therapeutic approaches to their work. While there are mental health teams who remain thoughtful in the face of extreme pressures and individuals who are naturally gifted and able to relate to patients in an open way, lack of training and support can leave professionals poorly equipped to deal with underlying psychological pressures inherent in the work. Training, supervision, and spaces for reflective practice are essential to support openness, thoughtfulness, and creativity. If this is not available, professionals may become closed off to underlying communications and overtaken by a belief that a patient's behaviour can be managed without being understood. The danger is that care then becomes dehumanized, mechanistic, and formulaic.

Effective mental health work depends on professionals' willingness and ability to be disturbed by patients while maintaining a professionally balanced view. However, establishing a therapeutic relationship with patients is complex and may itself be prone to false alliances, deceptions, and denial. These illusions and denials emanate sometimes from the patient, sometimes from the mental health professional, and sometimes from within the mental health system. Clinicians need a model for trying to take in and understand their patients' communications and suffering. Good practice depends upon practitioners' ability to use themselves and their own experience as a clinical tool. A psychoanalytic approach provides a model of the mind that allows for understanding both unconscious and conscious communication. It also provides a model for thinking about the relationship between the patient's internal and external worlds as expressed through the transference and countertransference.

CHAPTER ONE

Theory in practice

In this chapter, I outline some of the Freudian and Kleinian theories that I have found useful when thinking about clinical care in mental health settings, whether in direct work with patients or in teaching and supervising frontline staff. I also provide vignettes to illustrate the theory in clinical practice. In consultation and supervision, the skill is to introduce theory in a way that is relevant to mental health professionals' work. I have found that live supervision of a clinical case is the most effective way of bringing the concepts to life. It is important to stress that we all employ psychic defences in order to protect ourselves from overwhelming psychological pain and anxiety. Indeed, these psychic defences are essential for healthy functioning. However, there are problems when overwhelming psychological turmoil or conflict drives the individual to employ primitive defences in a rigid way.

Freudian and Kleinian theories

The transference and the countertransference

Freud (1895d, p. 253) discovered the transference phenomenon early in his work. He described the way the patient transfers repressed feelings and desires from childhood onto the therapist in the here and now. Initially Freud thought that the transference was an obstacle to therapy; however, he later discovered that the transference could throw light on deep-seated and repressed childhood conflicts. Patients develop powerful transferential feelings towards the professionals and carers responsible for their treatment. Professionals need to be sensitive to the meaning these roles carry for patients. It is important for them to try to·tune in to the patients' transference towards them, because this can convey meaningful insight into the nature of early relationships and underlying difficulties.

> At short notice I had to cancel the appointment of Ms B, a 30-year-old patient who always felt she had been a disappointment to her parents. She was born after her mother miscarried a boy, and she believed her mother would have preferred the miscarried baby to her. Ms B arrived at the next session saying that she nearly had not come, as she had assumed the cancellation meant that I no longer wished to see her, and she believed that I would feel that the therapy was a waste of my time. In her phantasy, she thought I would have preferred to see a more satisfying male patient.

Freud first described the term "countertransference" to denote the patient's impact upon the therapist's unconscious mind (Freud, 1912b). This idea was developed by Heimann (1950) to explain and make use of the therapist's feelings towards the patient. Her idea was that the patient generated feelings in the therapist that were responses to the patient's transference feelings. Money-Kyrle (1956) also developed this theory by differentiating between normal and abnormal countertransference. In normal countertransference, therapists take in the patient's experience and identify with it in a subjective way. Therapists then separate from the patient's subjective experience and objectively examine the interaction before deciding on an interpretation. In many ways, it is true to say that therapists are having a conversation with themselves before talking to the patient. In abnormal scenarios, therapists may have difficulty separating themselves from identification with their patients and react by treating the patients as if they were a damaged aspect of themselves.

Klein worried that this development could lead to wild analysis as analysts might attribute ideas and feelings to the patient for neurotic reasons of their own. Hanna Segal (1977) wrote that the countertransference was the best of servants and the worst of masters. She, too, emphasized the need for therapists to be cautious in attributing feelings in themselves to the patient. One of the functions of psychoanalytic supervision is to provide the space to explore therapists' or mental health professionals' emotional responses, to see how much light they shed on projective processes going on between them and the patient.

> Mr C, who was in his late thirties, was plagued by a feeling that he was not working hard enough. He was determined to gain promotion at work because he saw this as a way of triumphing over his sister. Mr C had always felt that his sister was the favourite and got the support of their parents at his expense. He came into the session, sat down in the chair, and after a few minutes' silence said: "Look, I can't afford to sit here wasting my time. If you haven't got anything helpful to say, I'm going to leave." My immediate response was to feel guilty, as if I had not been working hard enough or fast enough, leaving the poor patient suffering with anxiety about the threat of failure. After a pause, I began to find the space to separate myself from the effect of the patient's communication and think that this must be what it was like to be the patient: constantly feeling that he was never doing enough and that if he didn't keep himself under considerable pressure to work and progress then he would fail, his sister would triumph, and he would be unloved and unlovable.

The paranoid-schizoid and depressive positions

Klein described the healthy infant's dependence upon the mother for sustenance, care, and love in order to support the development of a strong ego and sense of self. When the infant feels safe, it feels that it is in the presence of an "ideal" loving mother and has loving feelings towards her. The "ideal" mother is internalized by the infant in a loving way and forms the basis of the infant's ego. However, when the infant feels anxious, in pain, or neglected, it feels that it is in the presence of a "bad" threatening mother who fails to provide protection and care. Aggressive feelings towards this uncaring "bad" figure then further threaten the infant's ego and sense of security. In order to protect the ego and any residual good feeling, the infant projects these aggressive feelings towards the "bad" mother out into the external world. These aggressive feelings are then felt to reside outside the object in the external world and are always threatening to return. Klein described the way the infant internalizes the good object it depends upon for life, in order to protect it, while projecting the bad threatening object into an object in the external world. The bad object is then attacked and treated as a threat that needs to be kept outside; this is known as the paranoid-schizoid position (Klein, 1935). The psychic defences used in the paranoid-schizoid position include splitting, projective identification, denial, and idealization.

> Early in the morning I sat down on the train opposite a man holding a can of strong lager, and he looked drunk. I glanced at him in passing. He seemed to be waiting for me to look at him. He became aggressive—"What the f*** are you looking at you c***?"

In this instance, the man has split off and projected his conscience into me, so that he is free to enjoy his inebriated state, free of conflict and questions. I then become his conscience, looking at him in a moralistic and judgemental way and asking him questions like "What are you doing, drinking at this time in the morning while everyone else is going to work?" He then attacks me in a paranoid way, in order to get rid of the questions and the critical thoughts. So here we have the man splitting off part of his mind and then projecting this elsewhere, out of his mind, hence "paranoid-schizoid".

Over time, as ego strength develops, the infant begins to lessen the split between the loved "ideal" mother and the hated "bad" mother. Indeed, the infant starts to recognize that the aggressive and loving feelings are both directed towards the same mother. The ideal object/mother is given up and replaced by the "good" mother. At the same time, the infant begins to realize that it is dependent on the good mother for sustenance and life. Faced with the guilt and subsequent realization of its dependency upon the "good" mother, it internalizes the "good" mother object in order to protect her from aggressive attacks. The infant mourns the loss of the ideal object mother; Klein called this state of mind the "depressive position".

In a psychotherapy session, a young woman who persistently harmed herself was suddenly aware of the fact that she had done tremendous damage to her body and her mind. During this session, she bent forward in pain and, in a way that conveyed her pain and anguish, said, "I can never repair the damage I have done to my body." She went on to say that she hoped she could stop self-harming because she still had a mind that had things to offer, and she would like to get on with her work.

In this instance, we can see how the young woman becomes aware of the damage she has done, which is irreparable, and this leads to sadness about the loss. At the same time, she is able to stay with the sense of loss, resist the temptation to get back into further acting out, and express a wish to protect the functioning part of her that is not damaged.

Manic defences against persecution and guilt

Klein also recognized that guilt and depression can lead to a regression into a manic state of mind, in which the infant tries to deny its dependence upon the object by denigrating the object and employing mechanisms of triumph.

Ms D, a 25-year-old patient with manic-depressive psychosis and a previous history of psychiatric admissions, was being seen in once-weekly psychotherapy. She had been stable for a number of years and was due to get married to the supportive man she had been living with. Her breakdowns had been precipitated in the past by casual affairs with men. These men had several characteristics in common: they were macho, good-looking, and sexually interested in her but not interested in other ways. Historically these affairs were often the precursors to manic breakdowns, during which Ms D would damage her relationships, self-esteem, and bank balance. Several weeks before a break in the therapy, Ms D told the therapist that she was sexually frustrated with her fiancé and had become attracted to a man who said he had been a member of a local gang and talked about killing men, which she found exciting. As the therapy break drew closer, she said that she was increasingly fantasizing about the violent man and planned to see him the following week. At the same time, Ms D also said she was worried about the forthcoming break in the therapy, which made her feel her therapist was worn out by her and needed a long rest to recover his strength. She had a similar worry about her fiancé, who, she complained, did not like sex as much as she did.

Ms D felt threatened by feelings of vulnerability and would turn to manic aspects of her own mind in order to triumph over underlying feelings of sadness and loss. As the marriage and the break approached, she worried that these ordinary, supportive men were not going to be able to provide the manic excitement she relied upon in order to triumph over her underlying feelings. Ms D was driven to distance herself from her underlying difficulties by starting an affair with an omnipotent, phallic man. The violent macho man represented Ms D's shift into a manic state of mind, in which excitement and violent psychic states triumphed over feelings of weakness, vulnerability, anxiety, sadness, and loss.

Reparation and manic reparation

Klein (1929) described reparation as the impulse to repair phantasied attacks on the object. Klein believed that reparation was central to all creativity, as individuals want to make amends for their attacks on the object through a creative act. Some reparative acts may take place in concrete external reality, while others are related to internal changes. As the object is symbolically repaired by the creative act, the ego is strengthened.

> A 28-year-old woman with a long-standing grievance towards her single mother for being overbearing came into therapy complaining that she could not establish a life of her own, as she felt this would be at her mother's expense. After some time in psychotherapy, she began to develop a capacity to put herself first and bear the guilt involved in developing a life of her own. Just before one Christmas break, she told me she felt guilty, because she had told her mother that she had decided to go to her new boyfriend's parents for Christmas rather than spending it with her. She said that she felt her mother was really hurt, but she was determined to put her wishes first and bear the feeling of guilt. A few months later, she told me that she and her boyfriend had decided to move in together, and she went through a similar feeling of guilt. She went on to say that she had just started playing the violin again, having not played since the age of 14. She started to cry as she remembered the pleasure that her violin playing as a child had given both her and her mother. Her mother had encouraged her to play the violin when she was younger, but she had given it up in her teens in a rebellious tantrum.

We can see in this example the way the psychotherapy helps the patient separate from her mother and bear the guilt of putting herself first. This allows the patient to give up her stance of masochistic but resentful compliance. She is subsequently able to rediscover a pastime that gave them both pleasure when she was younger. In this way she is able to bear the guilt of separating from her mother while rediscovering a warm and passionate relationship between herself and her mother, represented by the violin playing.

In contrast to reparation, which involves the experience of guilt, manic reparation employs omnipotent and manic defences in an attempt to repair the damaged object. The attitude towards the object often involves control and triumph rather than genuine remorse.

A patient in the early stage of therapy had a habit of going into loud and violent verbal outbursts when she was upset. As we came to the end of the therapy, she worried that she had damaged me through her verbal attacks and that I would be very keen to see the back of her.

Several weeks before the end of the therapy, she told me a dream. In the dream, *I was speaking at a prestigious conference, and she was in the audience with a friend. At the conclusion of my paper there was a long ovation, and the patient remembers feeling superior to her friend.* I said I thought she wanted to end her treatment with a long applause, admiring me as a figure of eminence, as this allowed her to feel that she had received a superior therapy and therapist, which would help to keep her above more ordinary feelings of anger and disappointment as well as gratitude and feelings of loss about me as her therapist. However, she worried that she could not protect anything ordinary from her criticism and contempt. She then said she remembered at the end of her dream seeing *a beggar on the steps of the university. He was dishevelled and unkempt but also bald, and he reminded her of me.*

In the example above, we can see the way the patient wishes to deal with her anxieties about the damage she may have done to me during the therapy by flattering me. However, the dream also reveals her triumphant feelings in relation to her friend. In this way, she tries to triumph over ordinary feelings of anger, disappointment, as well as gratitude about the end of the therapy. The association to the beggar on the steps of the university reveals the underlying anxieties about the damage she fears she may have caused me by her verbal attacks.

Projective identification

Klein used the term "projective identification" to describe a mental process in which the person gets rid of unwanted psychological knowledge or perceptions, while putting pressure on objects to conform to his omnipotent view of the world (Klein, 1946). Klein also outlined the infant's fluctuations between the disintegrated states of mind—the "paranoid-schizoid position"—and the integrated states of mind—the "depressive position" (Klein, 1935). In the paranoid-schizoid position, the infant's loving feelings for the mother are kept separate from its hateful feelings; thus, the ego and the object are split between an idealized, loved object and a denigrated, hated object. The infant then acts towards the external object as if it were identified with the element projected from the infant's mind.

> Mr E, a patient I saw in psychotherapy, had very little tolerance of his emotional difficulties and usually wanted to get away from the problem once he had told me the facts. Indeed, when I tried to think with him about the difficulty he had raised, he frequently said that he was bored with the subject and wanted to move on.

> Mr E started one session by telling me about an upsetting argument he had had with his girlfriend over the weekend. I paused for a minute, thinking about his communication, and within a few seconds he asked me if I was bored. In a split-second, the intolerance of his difficulties had been projected into me, and in his mind I had become the one who can't stay with an emotionally upsetting problem.

The depressive position comes about when the infant is able to reduce the split between the good mother and the bad mother and begins to realize that the mother he hates is the same as the mother he loves. This process of integration demands that the infant has internalized a good object capable of bearing painful emotions as well as being able to reflect upon the meaning of those emotions.

The depressive position and loss of the ideal mother coincides with the emergence of the oedipal situation as the infant becomes aware of a third object—often the father. Knowledge of the parents' sexual relationship creates feelings of curiosity as well as jealousy and loss. The triangular relationship between the parents and the child closes a psychic space and provides boundaries around the child's experience of itself. On the one hand, patients have an experience of their mother taking in their subjective experience, while, on the other hand, they are aware of a third object—the father—who is looking at the child's relationship with the mother from a different point of view. This model allows the integration of the infant's subjective experience of being understood emotionally by the mother with the objective experience of being thought about by the father from a separate point of view. This form of triangulation is necessary as it provides a space in which the object can be thought about in its absence, and it paves the way for symbolic thought (Britton, 1989).

Symbolization and concrete thinking

Segal (1957) built on Klein's ideas by describing the difference between a symbolic representation and a symbolic equation. In the case of a symbolic representation, there is an acknowledgement of the difference between the symbol and the object being symbolized. Thus, in saying, "I've got butterflies in my stomach", we are describing a sensation of things fluttering around in the stomach caused by anxiety or apprehension. We don't actually mean we have butterflies in our stomach.

In the case of a symbolic equation, on the other hand, there is no differentiation between the symbol and the object. This gives rise to what we mean by concrete thinking—using words (symbols) as if they were the thing (object) itself. Patients in psychotic states of mind often think concretely and thus might hear the individual saying "I have butterflies in my stomach" as a statement of fact rather than a symbolic communication. Thus, in a symbolic equation the statement "give me a minute" is interpreted literally as 60 seconds, rather than the symbolic meaning of the idea, which is "allow me some time". In order to maintain the difference between a symbolic equation and symbolic representation, the subject needs to be supported in establishing a psychic separation from the concrete object.

Container and contained

Bion (1962a) described the infant's dependence upon the mother for emotional and psychological as well as physical development. He described the way the infant's immature ego, overwhelmed and unable to process raw psychic experiences, evacuates and communicates these through noises, looks, and bodily movements. The mother takes in these raw experiences, before using her capacity to empathize and think about the infant's state of mind. Bion described this as the mother's capacity for reverie. In order for this process to work, the mother needs to be able to be affected by the communication without being overwhelmed. She conveys her understanding of the communication through her actions and loving attitude. Thus, the mother's ability to "contain" the infant's raw emotions helps to convert them into food for thought, which the infant can now internalize and digest. This gives the infant the feeling that it is being cared for by a figure that understands its feelings.

> A psychotic young man, agitated and threatening, was shouting and screaming at some staff in the corridor of a large mental hospital. Initially the staff talking to the man were kind and calm, but they tried to get him to do things: "Why don't you come in here?". . . "Why don't you take this to calm yourself down?" These reasonable requests lead to the man becoming more agitated and defiant: "Why don't you all leave me alone? I'm going to break you all!" In addition to calling the psychiatric emergency team, the ward manager had also called a well-known nursing assistant called Roberts. Roberts, an extremely large man, rarely felt threatened in physically threatening situations, and he had a reputation for calming down even the most psychotic and agitated patient.

> Roberts arrived, walked purposefully towards the patient, and started talking to him in a calm but confident manner. He acknowledged the fact that the patient was upset about something and invited him to stay where he was and tell him what was bothering him. Roberts's calm concern was evident in his attitude and his voice. As this went on, the patient seemed to

change from an agitated, aggressive, psychotic man into a much smaller, frightened, distressed child. The whole atmosphere changed, and the crisis began to dissipate.

Roberts's experience in dealing with these situations and his physical size meant that he was able to take in the patient's disturbance without feeling overwhelmed with anxiety about the physical threat. He was also able to realize that behind the threats and boastful claims of what the patient was going to do to the staff, the patient was in fact a frightened man. Thus, Roberts was able to contain the patient's extremely disturbed and threatening state of mind. This made the patient feel that he was with someone who was not terrified or alarmed by his communication but was, rather, someone concerned for him and able to both withstand and understand him.

The oedipal triangle and symbolic thinking

Freud (1950 [1892–1899], Letter 71, p. 263) coined the term "Oedipus complex" to described the way, at the age of between 3 and 5 years, the boy harbours rivalrous feelings towards his father as he phantasizes that he would like to murder his father while taking his father's place as his mother's partner. In the original myth, Oedipus unknowingly murders his father and marries his mother. Britton (1989) describes the importance of the oedipal situation in supporting thought and the development of symbolic thinking. He emphasizes the importance of the third object (psychically the father/partner) in supporting the mother-and-infant couple, while also providing room for separation and thought. The triangular situation provides a structure for thinking and helps to prevent collapse into concrete thinking or enactments.

Teams that treat patients whose clinical condition is accompanied by disturbing psychological states of mind can need the help of an external supervisor. For example, in mental health settings, patients with borderline personality disorder often get under the skin of staff, while those with antisocial personality disorder can induce sadistic responses from staff. These patient groups can have a profound impact upon staff, which can undermine the team's capacity to contain their patients. By acting as the third point in the nurse–patient–supervisor triangle, the supervisor can provide an appropriate space for thinking about the psychological impact of the work and reduce the pull towards re-enactments (Evans & Franks, 1997).

In order to develop and maintain a balanced approach, clinical staff need settings and structures that help them to digest the anxieties and pain involved in their work. Support needs to be provided through clinical discussion, reflective practice, and good management. On the one hand, these opportunities can help the nurse separate from the effect of the patient and restore an objective clinical approach, while, on the other, staff who have become hardened are helped to reflect more on the emotional impact of the clinical contact. These organizational reflective structures act like Bion's maternal reverie and support nursing staff through a process of containment, followed by separation and thought. Thus, reflective practice helps nurses to maintain the difference between the patient as a symbolic representation of their own damaged figures and a concrete symbolic equation with them.

The psychotic and non-psychotic parts of the mind

Bion (1957) described the way a split can develop between a psychotic and a non-psychotic part of the mind. The psychotic part hates any knowledge of psychological pain, vulnerability, damage, or weakness and tries to solve complex emotional problems through concrete physical actions, and it attacks the part of the mind that is capable of experiencing psychological pain and conflict—the non-psychotic part. The ego's capacity to perceive and think is attacked, fragmented, and projected into the external world. Thus, individuals feel that the external world contains fragmented elements of their own mind that threaten to violently re-enter the personality.

Bion described these objects in the external world, which contain elements of their own mind, as bizarre objects. Thus, patients in a psychotic state of mind may project their capacity to see into external objects, such as a clock. They then believe that the clock, which now contains an element of their capacity to see, is looking at them. These external objects have a threatening and persecutory quality as they threaten to push themselves back into the patient's mind. Thus the clock, which symbolizes an awareness and observation of the passage of time, threatens to force its way back into the mind of a patient who remains unaware of the way time passes. The vacuum left by the fragmentation and projection of parts of the patient's ego is then filled with an all-powerful and all-knowing delusional system, which is an attempt by the individual to repair a fragmented ego, in order to provide coherence and continuity. Propaganda emanating from the psychotic part of the personality is used to deny the reality of what has happened to the ego. The non-psychotic part of the mind has the difficulty of dealing with emotional problems while being undermined and attacked by the psychotic part of the personality. The psychotic and non-psychotic parts of the patient's mind are in a dynamic relationship and wrestle for control. Sometimes psychotic patients will project the non-psychotic part of the ego, in order to free themselves from the pain of the conflict between the two parts of their mind.

A ward manager from an acute psychiatric ward presented the case of a 40-year-old man.

> The patient had taken his passport from the ward in order to withdraw some money from the post office. The previous week he had lost his bus pass, and the ward manager was concerned he would lose his passport too. On his return to the ward she asked him where his passport was, and, sure enough, he had lost it. She then asked the patient to remember his steps, in order to help find it, but the patient replied that he was too tired and could not be bothered. The nurse became irritated, saying to the supervision group that she often found herself running around picking up after this patient, who tended to treat her as a servant.

> The patient, the eldest son of a successful academic, had had a promising career in medicine before suffering from his first episode of mental illness at the age of 20 years. He had had placements in several mental health hostels, all of which

had broken down on account of the patient's superior and immature attitude towards community living and self-care. The ward manager said that this situation created a management problem: the patient was occupying a valuable inpatient bed, and she was under pressure to discharge him, but he showed no inclination to rehabilitate himself or take any responsibility for his treatment.

During the supervision discussion, we thought about how the patient's actions seemed to symbolize something important about his mental state. He projected the non-psychotic part of his mind into the ward manager who had responsibility for looking after him. The ward manager acted like a mother who follows her child around, picking up things that have been used and have been discarded once they have served their purpose. It would appear that until the patient was helped to develop an interest in his own identity, mind, and history, including the circumstances of his tragic and catastrophic breakdown, he would have difficulty taking any responsibility for the management of his illness.

The internal narcissistic gang

Rosenfeld (1971) developed the idea of a defensive structure that acts like an internal gang and offers protection from psychic pain, in return for loyalty. Any move towards help by healthy aspects of patients may be undermined and attacked by destructive aspects of their internal world. Although healthy elements of such patients may consciously wish to divorce themselves from the gang's influence, they are often unconsciously dependent upon the gang in subtle ways. Their healthy part needs help and support in its struggle with the internal gang and in its attempt to form healthy relationships with good and helpful figures in the external world.

A young woman with a long history of anorexia, who had previously found it difficult to engage with and make use of her therapy sessions, started to engage and make emotional contact with the therapist. After three months during which she appeared to be more available in the therapy and making progress, she retreated into a withdrawn, silent state of mind and started to lose weight. Eventually, after several sessions where the therapist attempted to take this up with her, she confessed that she was hearing a voice telling her not to talk to the therapist and not to eat.

The improvement in the patient's condition and her move towards life and dependency provoked the gang to re-establish its control over her by pulling her back into an anorexic state of starvation and self-sufficiency. Separation from the influence of the gang often leads to a negative therapeutic reaction.

Steiner (1993a) built on Rosenfeld's work by describing the development of a "psychic retreat" within the patient's mind that acted as a resting place from anxieties associated with fragmentation on the one hand and development on the other. He also emphasized the need for clinicians to respect the fact that patients will inevitably move in and out of their psychic retreats in the process of recovery and development.

Discussion

In this chapter, I have emphasized the relevance of psychoanalytic theory in relation to helping to explain and understand clinical situations in mental health settings. It is important to point out that we all rely on defence mechanisms and defensive psychic structures to protect the ego from being overwhelmed. However, there is a difference between psychotic and neurotic defences. Psychotic defences, based on splitting, projective identification, denial, and rationalization, involve a gross distortion of psychic reality, which interferes with the individual's capacity to test reality and respond to the demands of internal or external realities. More neurotic defences, such as displacement, reaction formation, isolation, undoing, or repression, involve only a partial distortion of reality. All of us revert to psychotic psychic defences from time to time when we feel overwhelmed. However, the fragility of the ego and/or the severity of the superego mean that some individuals find the frustration and anxiety involved in contact with internal and external reality difficult to bear. These individuals may become reliant on psychotic defences to protect their fragile ego from being overwhelmed. It is also important to acknowledge that these psychic defences can occur within groups and institutions. Indeed, increased pressure on groups and individuals may push them towards psychotic forms of defence in an attempt to deny reality.

CHAPTER TWO

Psychoanalytic supervision in mental health settings

Patients who suffer from a serious and enduring mental illness often need psychological, chemical, and sometimes physical containment. The types of setting that provide this containment and the balance of the interventions used will vary according to the patient and his or her level of disturbance at any given time. It should also be remembered that the patient's mental state is dynamic and changes in response to many influences, one of which is the clinical care setting. For example, patients in psychotic states may present as calm and controlled in a psychiatric intensive care unit but become more disturbed once transferred to a less intensive setting. Patients need to be cared for by staff who are receptive to their experiences and who are willing to take in the patients' communications. In order for this receptive capacity to be sustained in the minds of staff, they, in turn, also need to feel looked after and that senior clinical management take their concerns and feelings seriously. If staff do not feel cared for by management, this affects staff morale, and they tend to become more anxious and less psychologically receptive to their patients.

In this chapter, I outline how psychoanalytic insights can help mental health professionals in their understanding and management of patients. Staff can benefit from understanding the way these unconscious communications can draw them into responses and actions that bypass the development of meaning and understanding. It can also help to prevent staff from colluding with the part of patients' minds that wishes to deny their illness. This results in an increased risk of clinical decisions being made that fail to take the underlying disorder into consideration, exposing patients to the risk of relapse. It is equally important that managers understand these dynamics in order to look after their staff. I have found that psychoanalytic supervision expertise is much needed and, indeed, valued by frontline staff. However, it helps if psychoanalytic psychotherapists who provide the supervision have relevant clinical experience of the patient group.

Case examples

Coping with intimidation

A CPN from a mental health team presented the case of Ms F.

> Ms F suffered from anorexia and had locked herself in her flat in order to starve herself. She had a habit of hoarding rubbish until it became a health hazard and posed a threat to other residents, whereupon environmental health officers had to be alerted. Ms F telephoned the nurse and said that she felt suicidal and wanted to die. The nurse visited the patient at home, but Ms F refused to open the door, so the nurse conducted a restrained interview with the patient through the letterbox. The nurse said that she was worried about her and was going to talk to her general practitioner (GP) to arrange a domiciliary visit. Ms F threatened to take out legal action against the nurse if she spoke to the GP.
>
> A solicitor then telephoned the CPN to complain about her attempt to speak to the patient through the letterbox, saying that she "would take out a charge of harassment" and that the nurse was "interfering with the patient's human rights". Several days later the nurse received a letter from Ms F's solicitor confirming this threat and that she should not contact the GP

under any circumstances. The CPN said she felt she was unable to take any action in order to help Ms F, because she feared prosecution. The CPN thought she was losing her mind as, on the one hand, she had a duty of care and Ms F was clearly ill, while on the other hand, she was in danger of litigation if she took what she considered to be appropriate action.

Bion (1957) described a division in the patient's mind between the psychotic and the non-psychotic (or sane) part. The psychotic part of the mind hates all emotional contact, psychic pain, and meaning. This part of the mind uses violent projection in order to get rid of any awareness of painful conflicts or emotions. The non-psychotic part of the patient's ego has the job of thinking about neurotic problems and conflicts associated with emotional pain and meaning. The patient's mind may alternate between these two states in what Bion described as "the conflict, never decided, . . . between the life and death instincts" (Bion, 1957, p. 44). When the psychotic part of the mind is in the ascendency, it may fragment and project the non-psychotic part of the ego in order to undermine individuals' capacity to think about themselves in relation to reality (Bion, 1957). The vacuum left in the ego is filled with magical thinking based on omnipotence and omniscience, rather than reality testing.

In the case of Ms F, we can see how the sane part of the mind was being held hostage by the psychotic part. Although the sane part of Ms F made fleeting contact with the nurse to make her aware of her predicament, the psychotic, murderous part stepped in and attacked the contact. This was done by threatening the nurse with accusations of professional misconduct if she went against Ms F's wishes. The solicitor had also been coerced by propaganda emanating from the psychotic part of the patient and designed to undermine the nurse's role and authority. However, Ms F's sane awareness relied upon the nurse's resilience and her capacity to hold on to the bigger clinical picture. The nurse's gut reaction was to realize that the threats were part of the patient's illness and that the sane part of Ms F's ego had been taken hostage by the psychotic part of her personality. Indeed, we could see that the sane part of the patient's mind was only allowed very limited contact with the nurse, represented by the initial phone call expressing her suicidal feelings.

Ms F's behaviour left the nurse feeling trapped and caught in a dilemma: if she did nothing, her patient's condition would deteriorate further; if she acted, she would be accused of abusing Ms F's human rights. This feeling of being trapped gave the nurse an experience of what it was like to be in Ms F's shoes, as the sane part of her mind was being attacked by the psychotic part of her mind if she drew attention to the extent of her illness. The message from the sane part of Ms F's mind was undermined and weakened by the psychotic part, with its accusations and attacks.

We can see the way Ms F's mental state fluctuated, as the dynamics of her internal world changed. At one stage, the non-psychotic part of her mind became aware that she was trapped inside a murderous psychotic state that wanted to starve her to death. This sane part of her mind was then able to let the nurse know that she was afraid she was in the grip of the murderous part wanting to kill her through starvation. However, once Ms F had made the nurse aware of her precarious state, she withdrew back into the psychotic internal structure, denying there was a problem. The psychotic internal structure then insisted Ms F attack and undermine the helpful contact with the nurse by threatening her with legal action.

In discussion, the nurse said that she felt intimidated and trapped by Ms F's threat of legal action on the one hand, but she knew she could not leave the patient on her own on the other. The nurse said that she found the discussion helpful, as it enabled her to think clinically about the situation. She also realized she needed the consultant psychiatrist's support in standing up to the intimidation from the psychotic part of the patient. The nurse subsequently reported that she conducted a domiciliary visit with the consultant, who told Ms F that unless she complied with psychiatric care, he would be forced to request a mental health act (MHA) assessment. The patient agreed to comply, and the need to section the patient was avoided.

Thus, the supervision group were able to support the nurse in her difficult work with the patient by providing a space for thinking about the underlying psychotic process, which allowed us to consider the meaning of this anxiety-provoking and frustrating situation. Once we could think of the fluctuating influence between the psychotic and non-psychotic part of Ms F's personality, it was possible to understand her perplexing presentation. The supervision group was able to help the nurse separate from the tyrannical influence of Ms F's psychosis by restoring her relationship with her consultant psychiatrist. The restoration of the relationship between the nurse and psychiatrist formed an authoritative clinical structure that could withstand the threats and projections emanating from the psychotic part of Ms F's mind. (We discussed that the solicitor would also need some help to free herself from the influence of Ms F's psychotic propaganda.) Investigation of the patient's mind is an important part of good mental health practice, and mental health professionals need the authority and skill to carry this out in a humane way. The nature of psychosis means that destructive aspects of the personality, which hate any acknowledgement of need, may attack and undermine either the patient's sanity or mental health professionals' attempts to help. From time to time, the non-psychotic part of patients' minds may become overwhelmed by psychosis in a way that forces them to act out their destructiveness in a physical way, resulting in a threat either to themselves or to others. When this happens, the patient may need to be physically contained (under the Mental Health Act 1983) and treated with medication. These interventions are not a substitute for psychological care, but they may be necessary in order to safely care for the patient (Alanen, 1997).

Denial and rationalization

A ward manager from an acute admission ward presented the case of Mr G.

> Mr G, a 26-year-old male with paranoid schizophrenia, had been admitted to the ward several weeks previously under section, believing that he was Jesus Christ. The ward manager said that Mr G upset the other patients, as he tended to talk in an aggressive way and ordered them around. She described his sexually inappropriate behaviour with the female staff. Mr G talked to them in a sexually uninhibited way, as though he believed that female staff found him irresistible.

After several weeks, Mr G's behaviour began to settle down, and he appeared to be less aggressive with other patients, although he always acted in a superior manner. He requested a Mental Health Review Tribunal and was successful in his appeal against his section. The tribunal stated that although they agreed Mr G was ill, they did not think he needed to be under section to receive treatment.

When the ward manager presented the case to the supervision group, she said that she thought that Mr G's behaviour became slightly worse following the tribunal. He would lie in bed until midday, refusing to get up for groups or occupational therapy, and then leave the ward. The staff suspected that he smoked marijuana while out, as he was often more disinhibited upon his return to the ward late at night. Mr G would then sit in the day room and get into arguments with the night staff, as he sat watching television until very late. The ward manager said there were continuing reports of niggling rows with other patients, as he would talk to them in a high-handed manner, and staff said, "It was a miracle that none of the other patients had hit him."

The ward manager said that Mr G had been admitted four times during the previous three years. He would be brought to hospital on a section after being found naked, preaching to passers-by in the street. Once on the ward and on anti-psychotic medication, he would calm down. However, he invariably maintained a superior air and distance from other patients and staff. Mr G would then make a successful appeal against his section, and some weeks later he would be discharged. Several months after being discharged, he would tell the Community Mental Health Team (CMHT) that he did not require any follow-up. Several months after that, he would start preaching again, end up in an altercation, and be readmitted.

Once in hospital, the positive symptoms related to Mr G's psychosis were quickly controlled by the medication and containment provided by ward staff. However, the effect of his psychotic beliefs continued to influence his behaviour, and this was evidenced through his high-handed attitude towards other patients and staff. The removal of the section made it easier for Mr G to leave the ward and self-medicate on marijuana. This, in turn, had the effect of making him increasingly "spaced out", detached, and withdrawn. Although there was no real evidence of Mr G having any substantial insight into his condition, he was sufficiently aware of his circumstances to keep his psychotic ideas "quiet" when talking to the Mental Health Review Tribunal. Mental health professionals often report that patients put on their best behaviour for the ward round or tribunal. The patients' presentations in these formal meetings can be significantly different from the picture presented to the nursing staff on the ward.

We can see how Mr G was able to conceal the positive symptoms of psychosis for a short period of time and in response to leading questions. Although he did not talk about his delusions in an open way, the on-going influence of the delusional system was evident in his behaviour and high-handed attitude towards others. Mr G acted as if he were Jesus Christ, the son of God, and above the ordinary ward rules. Indeed, he expected ward staff to recognize his special status and provide him with what he wanted, without any need for acknowledgement or gratitude. The negative symptoms of his illness also caused him to withdraw from meaningful contact with himself and others.

Diagnosis can be an important clinical tool, as it helps with decisions about treatment and prognosis; however, when assessment is narrowly based on the current clinical picture and concentrates too much on the presence or absence of symptoms, it leaves out important information about changes in the patient's presentation over time. Lack of insight and the presence of negative symptoms are as important in the diagnosis of a psychotic condition as the presence or absence of positive symptoms. There is always a danger that mental health professionals withdraw from emotional contact with their patients in order to protect themselves from the psychologically disturbing impact of the work. This withdrawal sometimes takes the form of a rather mechanistic and formulaic way of thinking that excludes curiosity about the relationship between her clinical presentation and the underlying personality structure. Distinctions between illness and health may be necessary to help categorize the patient's presentation and issues concerning treatment and clinical responsibility. However, this thinking can also be used defensively, as diagnosis does not invite the clinician to link symptoms and behaviour with questions about the patient's underlying personality structure, history, and ways of thinking.

Patients in psychotic states of mind often want to get away from the "headache" of thinking about their problems, and they can develop a condescending attitude towards their difficulties as a defence (Sohn, 1997). They may project responsibility for themselves into the individuals or teams caring for them. Nurses and other mental health professionals have the job of engaging with patients' sane part about their illness and psychological difficulties. This relationship, which is based on the need for help and support, is in conflict with the psychotic part of patients' minds, which use denial and rationalization in order to cover up the reality of their illness and the fragmentation of their minds. Indeed, mental health professionals can become the target of patients' condescending attitude towards their own difficulties as the psychotic part of their mind tries to distance itself from any difficulties and/or any need for help.

In the example outlined above, Mr G withdrew into a drugged haze and detached state of mind, free from worry or concern about his situation. At the same time, the nursing staff became increasingly agitated about his detached and "irresponsible" behaviour on the ward, and the fact that Mr G showed no interest in his rehabilitation but came and went as he pleased, without attending occupational therapy or ward groups. This irritation came through in the presentation of his case as the ward manager described Mr G as "treating the ward as if it was a hotel".

A psychoanalytic approach to clinical work can provide a model for thinking about psychotic symptoms and the relationship between different parts of the personality. This can then help clinicians develop their curiosity and interest in their patients' minds. In a paper about psychotic processes, Lucas describes the way in which psychotic patients rationalize and deny their illnesses. He also illustrates the importance of clinicians being receptive to, and tuning in to, what he calls the "psychotic wavelength" (Lucas, 2009e). If teams start to discuss their thoughts and ideas together, they can begin to think about how to engage with the patient in a new way: this gives an opportunity to turn a psychotic monologue attached to a delusional system into a dialogue with patients about their minds and the way they think (Taylor & Lucas, 2006).

The irritation in the ward manager's countertransference was due to Mr G's delinquent attitude towards his illness and his high-handed attitude towards ward staff and patients. Although he knew when to keep his grandiosity quiet, his actions showed that his mind was still dominated by his delusional beliefs. In that state of mind, he was above ordinary considerations about how he was going to manage his life or the need to take some responsibility for his mental illness. Instead, he projected responsibility for worrying about this into the staff. It was as though he believed he was staying at a hotel on holiday, with paid staff to look after his every need. The projection of his anxieties from the psychotic part of his mind left him free to imagine he was communicating with God—a belief that meant he did not have to listen to the authority of the ward staff. In other words, he had his own omnipotent and omniscient version of reality, which blocked out any uncomfortable or painful realities. The non-psychotic part of his mind, which contained all of the anxiety about his capacity to deal with the demands of reality, was projected into the ward manager. This left a vacuum in the ego, which was filled by Mr G's psychosis. The grandiose mental state represented his psychotic belief that he had managed to triumph over the frustrations and anxieties associated with psychic reality

The significance of countertransference responses in the assessment of risk

The following presentation was made in a seminar on one of the educational programmes at the Tavistock Centre.

A primary nurse from a high-security hospital presented the case of Mr H.

Mr H, a 31-year-old man who had committed murder, had requested that he be referred on to a medium secure unit, and the multidisciplinary team was considering this decision. The nurse said he was worried about the request, as he believed that Mr H remained highly dangerous. When the panel asked Mr H what he imagined for his future, he said he would like to live an ordinary life in a flat on his own.

Mr H had been sentenced to prison in his late teens for the murder of an elderly man. Mr H's victim had been unable to protect himself and had been subjected to various sadistic acts over a number of hours. Prior to his prison sentence, Mr H had had a history of drug abuse and burglary, but not one of violence. While in prison, he started to hear voices commanding him to kill himself. After informing the staff about the voices, he committed a serious assault on another prisoner. Mr H was diagnosed as suffering from schizophrenia and was transferred to a high-security hospital.

The nurse reported that Mr H's father had left his mother before he was born. When he was 10 years old, Mr H's mother found his behaviour too much to handle, and consequently he was passed between a series of relatives. One particular uncle used to beat him on a regular basis for minor misdemeanours. Mr H became a bully at school and was eventually expelled for his behaviour.

At the time of the presentation, Mr H had been in the high-security hospital for nine years, and his stay had been largely uneventful. Indeed, the fact that he was so undemonstrative meant that he was often moved around the hospital, and throughout this time he was maintained on a low dose of anti-psychotic medication. The seminar asked the nurse why he was so convinced that Mr H remained a risk. The nurse said that Mr H sent shivers down his spine because he was so distant, cold, and aloof, and that despite the fact that there had never been any serious violence during his stay in high security, he also felt Mr H was an intimidating man, who kept everyone at a distance. I asked the nurse if Mr H had any delusional beliefs. He told the seminar that Mr H had never mentioned any delusions, but he added that it was difficult to know what was going on in his head. The following week the nurse reported back to the group that on further investigation in Mr H's notes, he had found out that when Mr H was first admitted, he was suffering from a paranoid psychosis. Part of his delusional thinking was that he had been put on the earth by God to murder anyone who was weak or vulnerable. The nurse also told the seminar that Mr H had never demonstrated any acknowledgement of guilt over the violence of his attacks on his victims.

We can see how Mr H identified with the intimidating and bullying uncle as a way of dealing with his feelings of vulnerability. The voices commanding him to kill himself when he was first in prison represented projected suicidal thoughts connected to a threatening acknowledgement of his guilt. This suicidal state, which threatened to break back into his mind, was then projected into his victims (Sohn, 1997). In the psychotic part he believed he could rid his mind from the threat of the suicidal thoughts by first projecting them in a concrete and wholesale way and then by murdering the recipient of the projections. The whole process was justified, in the psychotic part of Mr H's mind, by a delusional belief that God had asked him to put these vulnerable and suicidal men out of their misery. Thus, the grandiose delusion hid his feelings of depression and worthlessness. He concealed the whole psychosis through his air of cool superiority on the ward. Following the nurse's presentation to the seminar, he had discussed his concerns with the clinical team, but the majority of the team thought there was no evidence of psychosis and that Mr H no longer posed a risk.

Several years later, I was informed that there was going to be an inquiry into the care of Mr H, who had committed another murder. He had been discharged from his medium-secure unit and, while in an acute paranoid state, had murdered an elderly man.

We can see how Mr H was able to promote a picture of himself as a reasonable man who had neither a mental illness nor a history of serious violence. His distant and superior approach to staff and other patients represented a condescending attitude towards the concerns of staff regarding his illness and his risk to others. In his delusional system, he believed he was put on earth to attack and torture weak and vulnerable people. This protected him from any sense of guilt for the damage done, or responsibility for managing his illness and risk factors. The projection of his sanity and any sense of responsibility for his illness and risk factors meant that Mr H remained a considerable risk. The change in the security of the clinical setting and all the containing structures that had previously supported his functioning as an inpatient having been removed, his mental state deteriorated catastrophically.

In my experience, the influence of the clinical setting and support available to the patient are underestimated in decision making and in the assessment of risk. For example, many patients' clinical picture can change as they move from high dependency to admission or to outpatient settings, as the increase in responsibility also increases the persecutory anxiety, which, in turn, increases the likelihood of acting out. The loss of relationships with significant members of staff is often given little thought when planning discharge. When these issues are neglected, it leaves patients on their own with their feelings of loss and anxieties about future expectations. This, in turn, can herald a return to regressive behaviour, which may increase risk.

The assessment of risk is not an exact science, and all risk-assessment tools tend to produce a percentage of false positives. It is also easy to be wise after the event, but people who suffer from a serious and enduring mental illness can be unpredictable by nature. However, there may be some important lessons to be learned from the case of Mr H in relation to his assessment. Certain patients project different elements of their mind into different parts of the clinical team. These patients are particularly difficult to assess because the projective process, which temporarily rids patients of unwanted elements of their mind, may in fact help them to present a false impression of coherence and sense. This picture can quickly break down when there is a change in the clinical setting, as the patient loses the containing structure and the split-off projections come flooding back into the ego, causing conflict and disruption.

Patients who split and project are often sensitive to existing splits in the clinical team as they pick up on rivalries between individual members of staff or disciplines. They may also pick up on divisions between lower- and higher-graded staff in teams that are overly hierarchical. For example, the ward domestic often sees a different side of the patient from the one seen by the ward consultant. Patients may also tune in to the way different teams privilege the views of particular disciplines or psychological theories. In situations where a patient is able to locate and project into existing splits in the team, it may become a blind spot in their clinical assessment and thinking. For this reason, relying on any one particular member of the multidisciplinary staff or one assessment tool can mean that vital elements of the overall picture are ignored.

When working with patients in psychotic states of mind, the countertransference can be a very helpful clinical tool as it gets behind the patient's denial and rationalization (Garelick & Lucas, 1996). The problem for the clinician is that the patient can "hold things together" for the duration of a mental state examination or review tribunal and can use rational and logical thinking stripped of emotion that appeals to the clinician's logic. The countertransference can help the clinician to gain access to the patient's underlying emotional state. The countertransference is particularly important when assessing psychotic states of mind, as the level of denial and rationalization may mask psychotic states. Of course, the evidence of the countertransference cannot be used on its own: it has to be corroborated by other sources of clinical evidence. It is also an important component of risk assessment because it can nudge the clinician into thinking about the patient in a different way. Indeed, it should be remembered that a particular member of the team may be in touch with a suicidal or homicidal aspect of the patient. This sort of approach can alert the team to risks that are unconsciously pushed out of the clinician's mind by the patient's denials and rationalizations.

Nursing staff are in a good position to make an assessment of the patient's psycho-social functioning over time, as they are able to witness the patient "in action" during ward activities, as well as through their own interactions with the patient. However, exposure to this disturbance can leave professionals with difficult, undigested countertransferential feelings. When these feelings get lodged inside, it can make mental health professionals feel guilty or uncomfortable, caught, as they are, between professional ideals of being endlessly tolerant and caring and other negative feelings of irritation, fear, disgust, or even hatred. These feelings can be dismissed by the individual as too subjective and personal and therefore irrelevant. Thus, countertransference feelings and intuitions—gut feelings—may be treated as if they are the individual's problem and not relevant to the clinical discussion. Although this might be true at times, wholesale dismissal of professionals' intuitions or gut reactions can deprive the clinical team of valuable information about the patient at an unconscious level. Good team leaders of multidisciplinary teams take an interest in the impact of patients upon the team and individuals. Not only does this show an interest in staff, it also acknowledges that countertransference and intuitive feelings can be used as prompts to think about the clinical picture in different ways. While such feelings are not sufficient on their own to guide decision making, they can alert the clinician to unconscious processes and blind spots in the clinical thinking. For example, had the nurse been able to corroborate his feeling about Mr H's coldness and aloofness with other objective observations, he might have been able to influence the thinking of the clinical team. If the emotional impact of the work is excluded from the clinical picture, this may leads to resentment among team members, and vital evidence of the clinical picture may be missed.

Issues of confidentiality

In the next example, I describe how a supervision group discussion helped to free a member of staff from the effects of her countertransference, changed the attitude of the staff towards the patient, and allowed room for some freedom of thought. This change in approach also seemed to have a dramatic effect upon the clinical picture.

A newly qualified social worker presented the case of Ms I.

Ms I was a regressed young woman with personality disorder who had been on the ward for a number of months but showed no signs of progress. When I asked the social worker to describe the patient's history, she said that the psychiatric team was completely in the dark. Apart from Ms I saying that her father had sexually abused her, she refused to talk about her history, saying it was too traumatic. The staff team knew from the referral that Ms I had been cared for by various other psychiatric services over a number of years. However, Ms I was adamant that she did not want the team to contact these other services.

In the supervision group we talked about Ms I's wish to control the treatment setting by making the staff feel they would be betraying her if they contacted the previous services. She also said it would be traumatizing to her if they asked her to tell them about her history. In the countertransference, the staff team were made to feel that they would become the abusing father in the patient's mind if they went against her wishes.

Ms I presented in a traumatized, infantile state, where there was only one possible version of reality, and that was hers. She feared that any other views would completely destroy her version of events. Although I did not know the history, I thought she was like a baby who believed that parents could love only one child. It was as though she was convinced that the birth of a second baby would deprive her of the love she needed to live. Thus, on the ward she had to maintain a tyrannical hold on her version of events, which allowed no other version to emerge. Compliance with this demand allowed Ms I to stay in a baby-like state within the ward, while the source of her disturbance—the second baby— was phobically projected outside the ward. By going along with this, it was as though the staff agreed with the patient that there was only ever one version of events or that parents could only ever love one child. For Ms I, any alternative view would constitute a traumatic assault on her.

In the supervision group we discussed the need for a broader assessment of the patient, including her history, the history of contact with other services, and possibly even her estranged family. We also talked about the need for the social worker to talk to Ms I about her fears of being dropped and discounted as the unlovable child if other versions (of reality) came to light. Even if there were conflicting accounts of her history, it did not mean that the staff team would dismiss her.

Several weeks later, the social worker reported back to the group that, following a discussion with the consultant and the multidisciplinary team, a decision had been made to contact the patient's previous clinical team. The social worker said she had also discussed this issue with Ms I, saying that the team needed to gather more of a picture. Ms I became extremely agitated, saying that she was worried that other services would lie about her and present her in a bad light. As we had discussed in supervision, the social worker said to Ms I that although they were interested in what other services had to say about Ms I's history and her treatment, they also wanted to understand her version of events. The team had the job of trying to make sense of what different people thought, as all views may be valid or contain helpful perspectives. She reiterated that they were trying to get as complete a picture of the situation as possible, in order to develop a fuller understanding of the patient and her difficulties.

The team social worker made contact with Ms I's previous social worker, who reported on the patient's history in care homes. Ms I did have a history of disruptive behaviour, splitting, and making allegations of mistreatment. With the help of further discussions in the supervision group and gathering various pieces of information together, staff were able to establish a picture of a very vulnerable, traumatized, and deprived woman. Staff could also see that although Ms I did try to manipulate staff and services, this was mainly done in order to try to maintain some fragile control over her environment. A plan was made to place the patient in an appropriate hostel for care leavers. The clinical picture continued to improve, until the patient was appropriately discharged.

Mental health services are required to respect their patients' wishes with regard to their treatment and rights to confidentiality. However, problems arise when services adhere to their patients' requests and wishes in a literal or unquestioning way, ignoring the clinical needs of the patient. In the case of Ms I, the patient was controlling the staff team's method of gathering information in order to make a meaningful assessment. This meant that the different aspects of Ms I's clinical care were being split off and kept apart. Although patients' wishes should be respected, problems arise when their desires are confused with their needs. Mental health professionals need to feel free to explore the patient's difficulties by gathering the fullest possible picture as part of their mental state examination and risk assessment. In my experience, less experienced staff are, understandably, reluctant to challenge or overrule patients' wishes, because they fear being seen as authoritarian. In the interest of getting things right, they may also be prone to interpreting guidelines in a more concrete way than they were intended.

The discussion in the supervision group, and then with the consultant in the multidisciplinary ward round, helped the social worker to free herself from the effects of the countertransferential fear that she would be traumatizing an already traumatized patient if they went against her wishes. Instead, they were able to discuss the issue of her fears and beliefs as a clinical problem, thus changing a conflict into an opportunity for a clinical discussion with Ms I about the nature of her beliefs; for Ms I, there could be only one version of events, and any new version would destroy hers. This was like the idea that a mother could only have and only love one child. It was important to discuss with Ms I the idea that although staff understood this, it was not the only way of looking at things. Indeed, staff could hold different versions of events in mind without it necessarily meaning that one version of events automatically discounted another.

Discussion

Patients in disturbed states of mind often communicate in ways that put pressure on the recipient to act rather than think. Psychotic communications have the emotional register squeezed out, leaving a concrete communication that does not invite a symbolic response. Borderline psychotic patients also put pressure on their objects in ways that cohere with their internal model. This provides them with reassurance that the object contains those aspects of the self that they would like to register in the object. However, although patients may be putting pressure on the staff team to react in a preordained way, problems can arise if the patients' wishes are carried out without any clinical thought or examination of the meaning behind the communication. Clinical teams and managers need to understand and examine communications before any course of action is decided upon. Particular consideration needs to be given to which part of the patient is communicating, and with what purpose.

The first clinical example shows how the psychotic part of Ms F's mind tried to suffocate the part of her that wanted to get help, and then tried to stop the nurse from acting by threatening her with legal action if she went against the patient's wishes. However, the nurse had already registered that Ms F was dominated by a psychotic tyrant that threatened to starve her to death. Understanding the dynamic struggle between the psychotic and non-psychotic aspects of the patient helped the nurse to understand the fluctuating communications and enabled her to instigate a discussion with the consultant psychiatrist about the most appropriate course of action.

When staff respond to patients' concrete demands in a concrete way, they miss the underlying communication. For example, if mental health professionals, mental health managers, or Mental Health Review Tribunals listen to patients' wishes or complaints in an uncritical or unexamined way, they may collude with patients' denial of their illness. This can lead to the patient at some level feeling that the staff have lost touch with the nature of their difficulties and can make them feel less secure.

In the second clinical example we can see how Mr G is able to conceal the extent of his psychotic thinking for the duration of the tribunal. However, once the section is removed, the psychotic part of the patient's mind is free to reassert its hold, leading to deterioration in the patient's behaviour and mental state. The MHA section acknowledges the extent of the patient's psychotic state of mind. Although the psychotic part of the patient's mind might argue against the section, the sane part of his mind can feel reassured that the mental health system understands the extent of the problem that needs to be contained.

If patients are dominated by the psychotic part of their minds, their non-psychotic part needs the support of mental health professionals. This sometimes means talking to the non-psychotic part of the mind about the problem they have managing the psychotic part of the mind. It also means that from time to time patients may need to be detained under mental health legislation or treated against their wishes, if they are believed to be a danger to themselves or to others. Freud believed that the unconscious was timeless; although symptoms may seem to disappear, they remain in the unconscious part of the mind and may return from their repressed state at any moment—particularly when the individual is under stress. For this reason, it is best to assume that a psychosis that is not apparent might still be present, somewhere, in the patient's thoughts or actions. Patients may need professionals to keep different aspects of their personality in mind, even when they are not currently apparent.

In the third clinical example, we can see how Mr H managed to conceal the nature of his psychosis for long periods in hospital. The threat posed by Mr H was picked up by the nurse in his countertransference; however, unfortunately this did not feature in the clinical team's assessment of the case.

Patients who suffer from a serious and enduring mental illness need services that take a long-term view of their difficulties. They also need settings that offer psychological, medical, and sometimes physical support. Patients may move between different parts of the mental health system as they go through different stages of life and different stages of illness. The usual rules of confidentiality may need to be overridden by clinical need, as it is essential for services to communicate between one another. Patients also need teams that understand that patients may split off and project different aspects of their minds into different parts of the clinical team or system. If this is not understood, it can cause unhelpful splits between staff and or between different clinical teams, which may exacerbate the problems of understanding and managing the patient.

In the fourth clinical example, we can see the way Ms I tried to control the clinical situation by discouraging the team from contacting mental health services that had previously cared for her. The supervision group was able to point out not only the possible meaning behind this controlling attitude, but also the way it fuelled the patient's omnipotent attitude to the clinical situation. Patients who split and project may fear that the services or professionals may gang up on them if they are in contact with one another. However, the integration of the clinical picture is an essential part of good mental health work. Indeed, patients often feel relieved when the different professionals and agencies talk to one another. This reduces the patients' omnipotent control of the mental health system and can, in turn, help professionals to deepen their understanding of the clinical picture.

Mental health professionals can use psychoanalytic thinking to help them understand their patients and support them with their difficulties. This understanding can also help them to stay engaged and emotionally available to their patients, even in the face of bizarre behaviours or communications that may have the effect of discouraging interest (Martindale, 2007). Psychoanalytic supervision provides a model that can help staff to think about these different symptoms and forms of communication. More than anything else, patients who suffer from a severe and enduring mental illness need staff who are human, curious, and interested in them as people and willing to see behind the bizarre behaviours to the human communication that lies beneath. Psychoanalytic supervision in mental health settings can provide a clinical structure that supports clinical thought and enquiry, looking for the meaning underlying the patient's communications and supporting therapeutic factors in the patient–clinician relationship.

CHAPTER THREE

Being driven mad: towards understanding borderline states

Borderline personality disorder (BPD) is characterized by unstable interpersonal relationships and self-image, and there is often a pattern of fluctuation in mood from periods of confidence to times of despair. These fluctuations can be related to feelings of rejection and criticism, which can lead to self-harm or suicidal ideation. Patients with BPD also have high levels of co-morbidity and are frequent users of psychiatric and acute hospital emergency services. Borderline personality disorder is present in just under one per cent of the population and is most commonly diagnosed in young women. Although some people recover over time, others may continue to experience social and interpersonal difficulties to varying degrees throughout life.

From my experience of supervising and teaching mental health professionals in both inpatient and community settings, I have found that patients who are described as borderline often present the mental health team with one of their most difficult clinical headaches. Indeed, the term "borderline" is sometimes used in a pejorative way to describe a challenging patient, irrespective of the diagnosis. Mental health teams are frequently divided between those who think that the patient has been victimized and mis-understood by services and others who feel that the patient is manipulative and needs to be discharged because no "genuine" or treatable mental illness can be seen. In confidence, individual team members may say that they really do not like the patient or are "driven mad" by them and find them impossible to work with.

So, why are patients with borderline features so challenging, and why do they prove such a headache for mental health services? In this chapter, I aim to help answer these questions and discuss how a psychoanalytic approach can complement other treatment methods and provide a helpful model for thinking about these complex clinical presentations. Indeed, professionals' feelings about their patients can provide an invaluable source of information about the nature of the clinical problem. I also argue that "frontline" mental health professionals need appropriate clinical training as well as ongoing supervision to increase and maintain their psychological mindedness in the face of their patients' concrete communications. This type of support can help to reduce the risk of patients acting out, as well as that of professional misconduct. It may also lessen the number of damaging complaints against staff and the destructive effect this can have on the clinical team. Without this support, these clinical challenges can seriously interfere with patients' treatment, care, and recovery.

All the patients described in this chapter caused a mixture of strong feelings, including sympathy, confusion, anger, hopelessness, and guilt. Although these views were not expressed in formal ward rounds or recorded in clinical notes, evidence of their influence could be seen in the staff's attitude towards the patients. In supervision groups, staff might say that the patients were victims of mistreatment or, alternatively, might adopt a rather moralistic tone, saying, "The patient is attention-seeking", "manipulative", or "not mentally ill". Psychoanalytic supervision, by putting the transference–countertransference relationship at the centre of practice, can help staff think about the feelings aroused by the patients' powerful communications and digest these feelings in a way that makes use of them as clinical evidence, rather than discarding them as purely subjective and/or judgemental. It also helps to reduce the toxic effects of the patient's projections upon the clinician's mind, and this in turn helps to reduce retaliatory or manic clinical decisions.

Patients who have borderline features as part of their mental state can be difficult to understand, as they alternate rapidly between different states of mind—from coherent and apparently insight-ful, to dissociated and on the edge of psychosis. For instance, one patient I saw for individual treatment spent the morning working as a nurse on a busy medical ward and the afternoon as a patient in a different hospital A&E, having self-harmed or taken an overdose. Patients in this state of mind can be extremely sensitive to rejection, and any mention of "discharge from care" can lead to an escalation of acting out, regardless of whether the patient has signed up to the plan of action. Indeed, even the idea that the patient is progress-ing can provoke the most savage deluge of destructive behaviour, which can set treatment plans back by weeks or even months. The serious and sometimes violent nature of their acting out may force mental health professionals to take responsibility for their behaviour for periods of time. However, these episodes of crisis can be accompanied by demands from patients for their independ-ence and capacity to think for themselves to be respected. Mental health professionals are often bemused and irritated by fluctua-tions in patients' presentations: one minute they are expected to take responsibility for patients' self-harming behaviour, as if they cannot be expected to care for themselves; the next they are being accused by the same patients of treating them like children, as if they are incapable of looking after themselves. For instance, one patient would act out during the week to ensure the continuation of ongoing one-to-one observation, then ask for leave from the ward at the weekend.

This presentation can lead to professionals resenting the contra-dictory nature of the demands placed on them. Not surprisingly, staff and services sometimes back away from such patients and look to either placate them or discharge them on to another service, as they do not want to be left in the proverbial "firing line". On the one hand, staff may hide behind a defensive position in which they start to moralize about the patient questioning their treatabil-ity or clinical need—an argument often used to justify discharge while at the same time protecting the professional from feelings of guilt or failure. On the other hand, patients can also excite power-ful rescue phantasies, which can contribute towards incidents of boundary breaking and serious professional misconduct. Patients in borderline states of mind may be very dependent upon services, as they demand high levels of care and attention. At the same time they may be extremely sensitive to feelings of humiliation and/or rejection. Indeed, they can be critical of the care they receive and complain that the care is insensitive or abusive. In some ways they may, in fact, be correct in claiming that they are mistreated and/ or misunderstood, as the violent nature of their actions and projections often provokes violent reactions from others.

Patients in borderline states of mind usually have fragile egos that are easily overwhelmed by internal conflicts and anxieties. Their minds tend to be dominated by a rather persecutory superego that only supports the ideal self and is intolerant of imperfections. Their thinking is characterized by paranoid-schizoid behaviour and splitting between idealization and denigration (Patrick, Hobson, Castle, Howard, & Maughan, 1994), and they may make extensive use of projective identification—Melanie Klein's term for the way a part of the mind may, in phantasy, be projected into an external object (Klein, 1946; see chapter 1).

This fragile and persecutory internal state is always threatening to fragment the ego and its objects. When this happens, the patient may quickly feel overwhelmed by persecutory anxiety; this splits the ego into ideal and unwanted aspects of the self, which are then projected into others in an attempt to evacuate the problem. The violent, concrete, and wholesale nature of the projections is also designed to have an impact on the recipient of the projections. Indeed, patients in borderline states of mind require the object to act in ways that confirm that the projection has hit its target, as this provides reassurance that the unwanted aspects of the self now reside in the other. The evacuative and projective process is also often accompanied by actions that force the object to respond in as concrete a manner. This cycle of action and reaction can drive staff and patients into polarized positions, which keeps the underlying conflict or problem obscured.

In his paper "On Arrogance", Bion (1958) described patients in borderline psychotic states as showing evidence of a catastrophic breakdown in their relationship with the primary object. It is as if the maternal object has been unable to take in and digest the infant's preverbal communications. Instead of the infant internalizing a good object that helps make sense of raw experience and becomes the basis of a healthy ego, it internalizes an "ego-destructive superego"—one that hates all emotional links and experiences.

This sort of internal object persecutes the patient. This internal structure can then become part of a destructive narcissistic structure, which employs omnipotent manic defences that are designed to avoid, rather than face, internal and external reality.

> A patient with anorexia and borderline features complained that a member of the nursing staff (who had worked on the ward for a number of years and had an exemplary record) had behaved in an unprofessional manner when she accused the patient of slowly killing herself. The patient's condition had been deteriorating despite several admissions over a number of years. When the complaint was investigated, the nurse said that she had been upset and angry when she saw the patient smiling at her in a mocking way. The nurse went on to say that she felt as if the patient were undermining their attempts to treat and care for her, while she gradually got thinner and thinner. She confessed that she had walked downstairs to go off duty but then returned to the ward and told the patient that she was "killing herself". The nurse was reprimanded as a result of the complaint and moved to another ward, while the patient died of starvation a few years later.

In this example, the patient projects any concern about her struggle to separate from her suicidal relationship with anorexia. This leaves the nurse feeling responsible for keeping the patient and her desire for life alive. Having successfully projected these desires, conflicts, and anxieties into the nurse, the patient is then free to mock the nurse and her caring attitude. Through the smile, the patient communicates her contempt for the desires, anxieties, and conflicts concerning her life, which are now felt to reside within the nurse. In this state of mind the patient is wedded to the deadly omnipotence of the anorexic state, as she feels she triumphs over the pain and conflicts involved in staying alive. The nurse is filled with rage when she reflects on the patient's mockery of care and her sadistic attacks on life. She accurately perceives that the wholesale projection of the patient's desire and wish for life leaves her in a deadly relationship with her illness. The problem is that she feels so overwhelmed with anxiety about the deadly state and so outraged by the patient's contempt for life that she wants to force what has been so violently projected into her back into the patient. The patient then rightly accuses the nurse of assaulting her with psychic reality.

However, the nurse is also right to believe that the patient needs to be urgently reunited with the part of her that wants to stay alive. If the patient goes on projecting her wish for life into the staff, she will remain wedded to the anorexia. Staff may feel provoked and helpless when faced with the patient's relationship with omnipotent defences. This, in turn, can induce a wish to "save the patient" through an approach that relies on omnipotent treatment. In this case, the nurse believed that the patient needed to be confronted with "the truth" about her illness. However, the painful truth for both parties is that omnipotent defences cannot be cut out, denied, or magically removed, nor can the patient be forced to face reality. Instead, the patient needs the nurse and mental health team to understand her internal struggle between the part of her that can bear reality and the part that feels that she does not have the psychic strength to relinquish her reliance on omnipotent defences. Recovery will depend upon her capacity to separate herself from her ideal self and mourn its loss. This, in turn, will expose the patient to ordinary anxieties about living, which she may feel ill-equipped to deal with.

The patient's capacity to cope with the demands of psychic reality will fluctuate during the course of the treatment process, with periods of development followed by regression. These fluctuations in the patient's psychological availability are an inevitable part of the recovery cycle. This struggle exposes both the nurse and the patient to anxieties about the outcome of the treatment, and this can be difficult for both parties to bear. Rosenfeld (1971) described the way some patients develop an internal destructive narcissistic structure, which offers to protect the individual from psychic pain through the use of omnipotent and manic solutions. The patient described above developed a deadly relationship with anorexia as a way of triumphing over problems of dependency and loss. I have found that professionals use the term "borderline" to describe a feeling that the patient has managed to "get under their skin" and provoke so much feeling that they have lost the capacity to reflect on their experience and feel like pushing something back at the patient. With the help of training and supervision, nurses and other professionals can tune in to the patient's way of thinking, allowing for more contact and understanding. This can also help to reduce staff frustration and acting out. Although acting in may be an inevitable consequence of the powerful unconscious forces involved in communication between mental health professionals and patients, supervision and reflective practice can help staff separate from the effects of these communications and restore their capacity to think objectively. This can reduce the tendency towards escalation in enactments and acting out.

Clinical phenomena in patients who demonstrate borderline features

Paranoid-schizoid thinking

Patients with borderline features function on the edge of the depressive position. However, when faced with disappointment and loss associated with a failure to reach ideals, they can feel persecuted and retreat into paranoid-schizoid states of mind. Narrowly preoccupied by anxieties concerning perfection and failure, they lose their capacity to take a broad view of their own or others' abilities. Their minds become dominated by black-and-white thinking and rigid splits. They project unwanted aspects of the self into the object. The following material acts as an illustration.

A staff nurse from an inpatient unit presented a suicidal patient, Mr J, a social worker who devoted himself to his job.

Mr J broke down after failing to gain promotion at work. He said that he hated any form of weakness, as he believed that the world was divided between Class A (strong and powerful people) and Class B (weak and helpless people). He said that he hated himself for being admitted to hospital, as this put him in Class B.

Mr J's family were all members of a fundamentalist Christian church, and his father believed that you should devote your life to the care of others. In fact, the father insisted that the family move to a poor part of Europe to help less privileged people. This move left the family permanently on the brink of financial disaster. His father's church maintained a belief that on Judgement Day, God's chosen people would be lifted up into heaven, leaving all non-believers behind. In his teens, Mr J had begun to develop a mind of his own and rebel against his father's beliefs, as he realized that they caused considerable heartache to his mother and the rest of his family. However, this development led to anxiety, as Mr J began to think that that he would be damned as a consequence of his doubts about his father's religion. This anxiety increased when he left school and went to college. At college he began a relationship and became infatuated with a rebellious female atheist, who suddenly and unexpectedly committed suicide. Following the suicide, Mr J started to become depressed and began to think that his dead girlfriend would be sent to purgatory, as she was a non-believer. He then developed an idea that he was responsible for her suicide because he had failed to convert her back to Christianity.

The primary nurse said that while Mr J was very passive, he was also demanding of her time and efforts. She said that she often felt she was not doing enough for him and that therefore she must be doing something wrong. She said she particularly felt this way following holidays or days off. Upon her return to work on the ward, she would be met by several staff who would tell her that they were glad she was back because "her" patient had been acting up. She emphasized the feeling that she could never do enough for Mr J.

Although Mr J gave up his Christian beliefs, he internalized a split world of idealization and persecution—a world that mirrored that of his father's fundamentalist beliefs. In his internal world, there was a powerful father figure that demanded complete devotion to his way of thinking. Any questioning of the ideal state led to terrible fear of reprisal and punishment. Consequently, Mr J felt that it was dangerous to separate from his father's ideals and to think for himself. Thus, Mr J was caught in mental conflict: if he accepted the rule of his father and devoted himself in a subservient way to the selfless care of others, he would have to give up his own mind; if he rebelled against his ideals and came to his own conclusions, he was in danger of becoming a failure in his father's eyes and being punished, pushed out of heaven and into purgatory. This claustro-agoraphobic state of mind left him caught between claustrophobic anxieties of being trapped and crushed by his father's ideals and agoraphobic anxieties about losing his father's love, attention, and protection.

This internal conflict between Mr J and the primary nurse was externalized and dramatized on the ward. Through countertrans-ference, Mr J made the nurse feel that she was not devoted enough to him and was not working hard enough to prove how much she cared for him. In this way, he gave the nurse an experience of what it was like to be in his shoes, as she was claustrophobically imprisoned by Mr J's demands.

The supervision group was able to help the nurse to separate herself from the feeling that she had to provide ideal care or else she was failing the patient. She realized that she had internalized a persecutory aspect of the patient's internal world that had been projected into her via a process of projective identification. The more she tried to prove her devotion and care, the more trapped she and the patient became in a mutually idealizing psychic prison. In this way, the relationship repeated the patient's relationship with his father.

The supervision group provided the nurse with mental space to examine her feelings about the patient. It allowed her to escape from the narrow mental trap of her countertransference and restore her capacity to think about the patient in a more realistic and objec-tive way. This involved letting go of the idea that she was saving Mr J by rescuing him from his mental illness. The group could then use the nurse's countertransference as a tool for deepening their understanding of the patient's psychopathology.

Patients in borderline states of mind sometimes unconsciously split and project aspects of their own ego into their objects in a forceful way. This makes integration of the ego difficult. With these split-off parts of the self located in external objects, which then need to be controlled, patients have difficulty establishing a stable identity. They consequently lose a sense of themselves and what they feel and think. In order to achieve a sense of stability, they require their host-object to behave in accordance with the aspects of the self that have been projected. Thus, they try to control other people by pushing them into a position in which the other person experiences something on their behalf, or, alternatively, they manage to provoke others into a reaction according to a script they have laid down. This psychic structure is largely responsible for patients' demanding, controlling, devaluing attitude towards their object. It also helps explain their experience of de-personalization and de-realization. In many ways, the degree of control imposed on others is related to the degree of fragility and insecurity in patients' sense of self. This underlying insecurity is often successfully denied and projected. Rey thought that in many ways these patients are searching for a supportive psychological structure that functions like a "marsupial pouch" (Rey, 1994). The extent of projective identification means that patients may feel as if they are living in the object, and consequently they are unable to separate from the object.

Identification with powerful figures as part of a concrete magical solution and cure

Patients with longstanding psychological difficulties can fear that they are damaged and cannot be returned to a healthy state without the help of some magical and superhuman solution. In an attempt to repair themselves and others, patients sometimes develop a concrete identification with a powerful person or ideal—one sometimes with grandiose or manic elements to it—that is a sort of getting "into uniform". However, the identification may be unstable and may rapidly break down when things go wrong.

A CPN gave a presentation to the supervision group about Ms K.

Ms K was a 22-year-old medical student with a two-year history of suicide attempts and self-harming behaviour. The CPN said that she and the team were trying to get the patient back to her training, but each time Ms K attempted a return, she started self-harming and threatening suicide. Ms K was in the third year of her medical training and had just started taking medical histories from patients on a female medical ward, when she was overcome by thoughts of wanting to die. After a serious suicide attempt, she was admitted to a psychiatric hospital. Following her discharge, she tried to go back to her medical training but could not forgive herself for her illness and admission to hospital. After some time, the medical school said that they were going to suspend her training. Following that, her self-harming behaviour increased; she was hearing a voice inside her head telling her that as she had "failed to train as a doctor, she might as well kill herself, as there was now no point to her life".

Ms K said her mother always made her feel bad for any failure at school. Ms K's mother had suffered from post-partum depression after Ms K was born. The mother started to drink, and her parents argued during her childhood. Eventually her parents separated, and her mother's alcoholism deteriorated further. The CPN said that the team had tried everything to get Ms K back to medical school but feared that they would fail again. She also worried that the patient might then become an even greater suicide risk.

Many patients with "borderline features" have experienced disrupted early lives, with fragile or damaged parental figures, and have not had the emotional and psychological containment necessary for healthy emotional development. They may have little capacity to tolerate frustration or think symbolically about their emotional life and tend to split off and project unwanted or unbearable aspects of themselves. This splitting and projection further interferes with their capacity to test their perception of themselves against reality or to learn from experience as the process depletes the ego. Consequently, there can be a difficulty holding on to complex "depressive-position" thinking as they tend to become overwhelmed by persecutory feelings and demands that need to be met immediately. They tend to develop identities based on denial and projection of certain aspects of the self and idealization of others. This fragile structure then requires other people to act as hosts for unmanageable aspects of themselves.

I thought that Ms K's wish to train as a doctor may have been psychically related to her wish to cure her mother's depression and her own depression about her mother's illness. As a child, she had been made to feel that she was not what her mother wanted and that she was unable to improve her mother's mood. Consequently she set great store on training as a powerful and potent doctor who could cure patients of their illnesses and restore family pride. However, this belief quickly broke down when seeing the chronic nature of the condition of patients on the female medical ward reminded her of the chronic and depressing nature of her mother's condition, which could not be cured by her efforts to be an ideal daughter. Consequently Ms K collapsed into despair. Beneath her hatred of herself was a hatred of her mother, who had made her feel so responsible for her illness. Without the identification with the ideal and powerful doctor figure, she felt that she was surrounded by damaged aspects of herself and impotent to cure her mother.

During the supervision, we were able to discuss the pressure the CPN was experiencing to get Ms K back into medical training at all costs. It was as if the CPN agreed with Ms K's concrete belief that the only solution to her difficulties was to get back into her doctor's uniform, as otherwise her life would not be worth living. There was also the terrible persecution of time, because Ms K felt the nurse had to help her to get back to medical school as quickly as possible. Ms K hated the fact that she had already lost time on her journey towards becoming the ideal object. The CPN was made to feel that any time away from the patient was slowing up the process and robbing Ms K of the time and support she needed to progress. In the countertransference, the nurse was afraid of being judged by the same harsh and blaming figure that dominated Ms K's internal world, if she failed to restore Ms K to her ideal state. The nurse was also made to feel bad for having time of her own away from Ms K.

The supervision group was able to help the CPN think about her patient from an objective point of view, based on her experience as a psychiatric nurse. She was then free to challenge the patient's belief that training as a doctor was the only cure for her underlying feelings of depression and impotence. Ms K needed help in letting go of her need to be the ideal and magical figure who could cure everyone else's problems while neglecting her own. This would then allow her to begin to face her own internal difficulties, including her feelings about her difficult childhood, and to mourn the loss of her ideal self.

In a paper on reducing suicide, Caroline Taylor-Thomas and Richard Lucas (2006) warned that patients may project the dismissive attitude that they have towards themselves into mental health staff. The countertransference then affects professionals' perspective as they join patients in dismissing the seriousness of the problem. Taylor-Thomas and Lucas point out that clinicians may join in with patients' invitation to dismiss their behaviour as acting out and miss an underlying depression. As outlined above, Ms K put pressure on the staff team to get her back to medical school at all costs. The acting out and episodes of illness were treated as if they were a psychological blip rather than an indication of severe psychopathology.

Repetition compulsion

Repeated patterns of self-harm or destructive relationships, which often form part of the clinical picture, are symptomatic of a damaged and damaging relationship with the self. Characteristically, these patients' have had relationships with impaired, abusive, psychologically fragile parental figures, and this may impede their psychological development. These abusive and neglectful relationships are internalized and form part of patients' attitude towards both themselves and others. Inevitably, these patients re-enact their traumatic histories in their relationships with healthcare professionals and the healthcare system.

A primary nurse from a specialist inpatient unit presented a self-harming patient to the weekly supervision group.

Ms L had a history of self-harm and damaging relationships, and she had been admitted to a specialist unit for the treatment of her self-harm. The nurse said that the patient was due to be discharged in a month. However, her self-harming behaviour continued on a weekly basis and, in particular, after the previous two weekends. She described a pattern of the last two weeks in which Ms L would wait until the ward manager and senior registrar had gone home for the weekend before asking if she could be allowed home on weekend leave in preparation for her discharge (all weekend leave was supposed to be discussed and agreed with the multidisciplinary team during the week). The nurse said that Ms L was very persuasive and argued that she should be allowed home because she was preparing herself for discharge. The patient promised not to go near her mother's house, as these visits always provoked arguments between Ms L and her stepfather, followed by serious acts of deliberate self-harm. Ms L would subsequently return from weekend leave having visited her mother, argued with her stepfather, and cut herself, all of which left the nurse feeling responsible. The nurse said that she felt annoyed with the patient, as she felt that her trust had been abused.

The patient's father had left when she was very young, and her mother had started to drink. After some years her mother had met and married her stepfather. Ms L resented her stepfather's arrival, because she felt that she had lost her mother to him. In her mid-teens, Ms L had accused her stepfather of abusing her, and he was removed from the house for investigation. The allegations were not substantiated, and he returned to live with the mother for several years before Ms L left home. The patient lived a few miles away from her mother, and every time she went out on weekend leave she visited her mother, they argued, and she harmed herself. The patient had a repetitive dream in which *she was trapped in a soundproof room being abused by her stepfather while her mother was outside the room and unable to hear her screams.*

I thought the dream accurately described a repeated pattern in the patient's internal world, as well as in relation to the unit and the nurse. In the dream, Ms L was caught up in an abusive situation with a sexualized father figure split off from the mother of her mind. Thus, she managed to split the parental couple and pull the father of her mind away from the mother of her mind and into an abusive, sexualized relationship. This deprived her of a parental couple who could help her assess the nature of her difficulties. I think the mother who is deaf to her daughter's cries and screams represents the ward staff who seem unaware of the patient's relationship with perverse aspects of herself and her objects. This whole scenario was re-enacted with Ms L's requests for weekend leave, in which she would break the conditions of her leave by returning to see her mother and stepfather. She would then re-enact the original trauma in which she would try to split her mother from her stepfather by provoking a row. When her mother failed to side with her against her stepfather, she would harm herself as an act of revenge against her mother. Ms L's actions drew attention to the fact that she remained in the hands of infantile aspects of herself that wanted to dominate her mother and punish her for having a relationship with her stepfather. Her difficulty managing painful emotions meant that she would be pulled into actions in order to discharge her feelings rather than think things through.

In the supervision, we were able to think about the way the primary nurse was seduced into agreeing with Ms L's apparently reasonable request without thinking through the conflict with the care plan or the meaning behind the request. In this way, the ward was enacting the role of the mother in the dream who could not hear how involved Ms L was in a repetitive, abusive, sexualized relationship with herself and her objects. I also suspect the senior ward staff's absence at the weekend was significant because they had gone off and left the patient in the hands of junior staff, thus repeating her view of her childhood trauma as her mother going off with her stepfather, leaving her in the hands of a junior aspect of herself. We discussed the need for the nurse to talk to the ward manager and consultant about the patient and her concerns about the patient's ongoing involvement with infantile and perverse aspects of herself that wished to punish her mother for leaving her but also resulted in further self-harm.

Patients with borderline features are usually sensitive to any splits that exist in mental health teams; they may use these splits to act out in a way that then provokes reactive responses from staff, preventing the latter from seeing clearly the patient's underlying state.

Patients frequently present themselves as the innocent victims of abusive figures, and in some ways this must be true. However, this view denies patients' involvement with the abusive aspects of themselves that attack and undermine their need for help. In a paper on severe personality disorder patients in prison settings, Hinshelwood described the large number of patients who had been abused in the past and then either became abusers themselves or became self-abusers; this self-abuse often became a feature of their attitude towards help and helpers (Hinshelwood, 2002). He also highlighted patients' sensitivity to the personality and intention of their carers and pointed out that carers were prone to be split between those who were seen as indulgent and lenient and others viewed as harsh, judgemental, and punitive.

Attitude towards the body

Kernberg argued that many patients who go on to develop a BPD have experienced relationships with hostile, aggressive, abusive carers in infancy and childhood (Kernberg, 1975). These early relationships may be taken into different parts of the patient's mind and body where they continue their hostile relationship with one another. Patients can dissociate themselves from their feelings and sense of responsibility for their body or actions, developing a split between the mind and body. The mind then develops a hostile and uncaring attitude towards the body, which is mistreated and abused without any thought or feeling for the consequences. Thus the childhood trauma, with its dynamic interplay of abuser and abused, is internalized and enacted between the patient's mind and body. The patient then triumphs over psychic pain by attacking the self and creating horrified reactions in others.

A social worker presented a patient to a supervision group for community mental health workers.

> The patient, Mrs M, regularly visited the hospital A&E department after inserting blades into her vagina. Mrs M was an attractive woman who had been abused by her father and went on to become a prostitute. She worked as a prostitute for 10 years and described her twenties and thirties as a "nonstop party". Mrs M had several terminations of pregnancy and contracted various sexually transmitted diseases. She also developed a severe infection of her ovaries, which required an operation to partially remove them. In her late thirties she met a man and settled down. However, she was unable to conceive as a result of the operation on her ovaries. Several years later her partner left, saying that he wanted children. Mrs M had a great deal of difficulty coming to terms with the separation and started to berate herself for her history of prostitution. She

would get drunk, cut her face, and insert small blades into her vagina. She would then call the police to tell them what she had done. In discussion with the social worker, Mrs M said without any emotion that she could not forgive herself for having her pregnancies terminated.

The social worker was disturbed, perplexed, and irritated by Mrs M's presentation, as she would swing between a calm and rather distant demeanour when sober and highly disturbed behaviour when drunk. The social worker went on to say that he thought the patient was attention-seeking, as she did not seem to be either depressed or psychotic.

In the supervision group, we were able to discuss the way in which the patient blamed her face and genitals for continuing the abusive lifestyle of her youth, and the way in which she believed that her genitals were infected with badness and bad desires rather than babies. The attack on her face represented an attack on her beauty and sexuality, which attracted so much of the wrong sort of interest. The blades inserted into the patient's vagina represented the patient's attack on the abusive sexual relationships. This interest in her sexuality was in contrast to a lack of interest in the rest of her mind and personality.

We talked about the way Mrs M invited the social worker to dismiss her symptoms as attention-seeking and meaningless. This attitude then re-created Mrs M's traumatic childhood history, as the social worker took on the role of a parental figure who did not want the headache or worry of this disturbing patient. The understanding provided by the supervision group helped the social worker to reconnect with his feeling of interest and sympathy for the patient as he was put in touch with Mrs M's underlying pain and the extent of her psychological damage.

Bick (1968) described patients who became overly reliant on the skin to hold them together in a psychological way where there had been some failure of psychological containment. Although many patients who cut themselves deny the extent of their psychological damage, their skin and body is used as a concrete and physical record of their damaged internal worlds. The cuts represent physical evidence of the wounds that have been inflicted by the "battle of life", and patients who show their scars off are like soldiers who wear medals and need to be admired for their bravery in battle (Leslie Sohn, personal communication, 2005). Many patients use self-harm to assist the mind in breaking the link between thought and feeling (or cause and effect); this break also means that patients cannot learn from experience, and consequently the cycle of behaviour is repeated. In place of thinking, patients often rationalize and justify their actions.

Anxiety about patients' self-destructive behaviour can push the mental health services into taking over responsibility for their care, whereupon patients can become dependent upon that care. An unhelpful spiral of self-destructive behaviour and further care can develop, until patients are eventually detained under mental health legislation and put on continuous and close observations to prevent further self-mutilating behaviour. This situation frequently leads to a malignant regression, as staff are made to feel entirely responsible for protecting patients from themselves. Any attempt by staff to reduce the amount of one-to-one surveillance leads to further acts of self-mutilation and escalating self-destructive behaviour, which ensures that patients remain at the forefront of the staff team's mind. The morale and confidence of the staff affects the use of one-to-one observations. Mature teams who feel supported by their managers are more likely to trust the team's capacity to manage their patients without resorting to one-to-one observations, whereas less coherent or confident teams are more likely to keep patients on them. Consequently, staff may feel that they are being controlled by patients and tormented by their behaviour, which raises anxieties about risk, as well as hostility towards patients.

The special patient

These patients have often had traumatic lives, and they can enlist professionals' sympathies and wishes to help. In his paper "The Ailment", Main described some patients in a therapeutic community who were treated as "special" by certain members of the staff team (Main, 1957). These patients were successful in eliciting special care, which caused splits in the staff team. This can become a sadomasochistic relationship in which patients sadistically attack the staff's feeling of hope or responsibility by harming themselves. The staff may then, in turn, act out the sadomasochistic pattern as their treatment of the patient becomes dominated either by a moralistic belief that the patient is not worthy of treatment or sympathy and needs to be punished or, alternatively, by a manic wish to repair the patient at all costs (Evans, 1998). A team that is dominated by a moralistic attitude may resort to a rapid and ill-prepared discharge while accusing the patient of being attention-seeking, manipulative, or hysterical. They may rationalize their behaviour by saying that the patient is not psychiatrically ill and "turn a blind eye" to important aspects of the patient's psychopathology (Steiner, 1985). This, in turn, may lead patients to behave in dramatic self-destructive ways in an attempt to force staff to continue caring for them. Alternatively, if the team is dominated by a manic wish to repair, staff push themselves to great lengths to help the patient, taking on more and more responsibility for the treatment. The patient is given special allowances but is kept in hospital without a clear treatment plan. Staff often become demoralized by this situation and resent the patient for defeating their best efforts.

Discussion

Patients with borderline features have difficulties in dealing with the psychic contents of their minds and tend to evacuate undigested elements of their minds through action. Different parts of the patient are projected into different parts of the psychiatric team, and splitting abounds. Such concrete communications fill their recipients with feelings that either provoke concrete reactions in return or make staff feel that they cannot think clearly about the patient. With staff unable to think in a symbolic way about the meaning of patients' behaviour, they and their patients can get into an unhelpful cycle of action and reaction that prevents learning from experience.

In the first clinical example, the nurse, provoked by the anorexic patient's contempt for life, tried to force her to acknowledge her murderous attack on life; unable to contain her upset and fury with the patient, the nurse acted out by marching back onto the ward and confronting the patient. In this instance, supervision might have enabled the nurse and the clinical team to digest the provocative mockery and turn it into a thoughtful therapeutic intervention.

In many ways it is true to say that these patients draw and push staff into dyadic relationships dominated by projections, which affect the staff's capacity to think in an objective or imaginative way. The staff team may be split between those members of staff who have been chosen by the patient and those who believe that the patient has seduced members of staff into a collusive relationship based on denial. The reality is that some members of the staff team may be trapped in an identification with the patient as a victim of mistreatment.

In this example, the member of staff has become stuck in an idealized role associated with rescuing the patient from terrible misunderstanding and persecution, while staff who have not been chosen by the patient can become filled with a moralistic belief that she needs to take responsibility for her behaviour. In the first instance, the rescuer believes she can support the patient's positive attributes by encouraging her to split off and deny her relationship with destructive aspects of the self; the moralistic group, on the other hand, avoid being made to feel responsible for the patient's behaviour and progress by developing a view that the patient is in control of her behaviour and "knows what she is doing".

While there is a degree of truth in both positions, problems arise when these beliefs become polarized and fixed, because it interferes with real clinical thought. The different elements of the clinical picture, which are often fragmented and projected, need to be gathered together in supervision and multidisciplinary meetings, in the interest of trying to understand the borderline patient's underlying state of mind. The staff's capacity to think about and make sense of patients who present with borderline clinical features is a dynamic process, relying upon numerous factors, including the team's capacity to verbalize and integrate the different views of the patient. This is a potentially turbulent process, requiring a constant examination of the mental health professional's contact with the patient, within an atmosphere of curiosity and openness. It also means that staff teams have to tolerate doubt and uncertainty about their work.

In the second clinical example, the nurse had become identified with a rescuing figure who was going to save Mr J from his mental torment. The staff team fitted in with this arrangement by describing Mr J as "the primary nurse's patient" and very much leaving them to function as a couple. The supervision group was able to help the nurse to separate herself from the belief that she had to rescue the patient and to re-establish her relationship with the wider nursing team in the treatment of Mr J.

Patients in borderline states of mind project in ways that affect the object, and mental health professionals often complain that these patients "get under their skin" or "drive them mad". The nature of the projection also pushes the object to cohere with the projection, and staff are often nudged into a response that confirms patients' projections. Indeed, the forceful and concrete nature of the projections often provokes a knee-jerk response in staff, and an unhelpful cycle of action and reaction between patients and staff can develop.

Steiner (2011) outlined the way a certain group of patients were able to use emotive accounts of external reality in order to get the analyst to internalize and identify with damaged aspects of the patient's self. The sense of being overwhelmed by internal damage would nudge the analyst into a position where he gave up the limitations of an analytic approach, in which he searched for symbolic meaning, in preference for a more active role in which he would subtlety advise and mould the patient's behaviour. Problems would emerge when this omnipotent approach broke down during breaks and separations.

Regular psychoanalytic supervision helps staff to process their feelings about their patients and also to examine the transference and countertransference relationship. The supervision group can help mental health professionals separate from the effect of projections by turning a dyadic relationship into a triadic one as the supervisor or group forms the third point of a triangle. The triangle provides space for an objective examination of the clinical picture, which includes the staff's subjective view. This type of objective examination helps to provide some psychic space, which frees members of staff from the narrow psychic state created by the subjective dyadic relationship that often develops in the treatment of patients with BPD. This triangular space also creates room for staff to think in an imaginative way about the underlying meaning of the communications and re-establish their capacity for symbolic thought.

In the third clinical example, Ms K believed that she had to train as a doctor in order to cure the damaged internal and external mother that persecuted her. The CPN needed help in separating herself from Ms K's belief that the desire to train as a doctor would enable her to triumph over her difficulties. The patient could then be helped to separate herself from her fanatical desire to cure her mother of her depression. This would involve her relinquishing her compulsive desire to manically repair her mother through her training and thus accept a more realistic assessment of her capacities and limitations.

It is also important in the treatment of borderline patients to establish a long-term view, which takes account of patients' underlying fragility. Individual episodes of acting out need to be seen within the context of the overall clinical picture and include an assessment of the borderline patient's personality structure. Psychoanalytic supervision, by developing a long-term view in this way, can also help staff teams to integrate clinical facts about their patient's history and personality structure with the current clinical picture. Although knowledge of patients' history will not necessarily prevent these re-enactments, forewarned is forearmed, and knowledge of the transference and countertransference may help staff tolerate the effect of the virulent projections. It can also help to address adverse countertransferential responses.

In the fourth clinical example, Ms L's dream represents a repetitive and perverse sadomasochistic relationship with her mother and stepfather. In the dream, she is involved in an abusive erotized relationship with the stepfather in her mind, while the mother in her mind is accused of being deaf and uninterested. In many ways, Ms L has failed to mourn the loss of her relationship with her mother, and she harbours resentment and grievance about the arrival of the stepfather. The dream represents an erotized sadomasochistic relationships used to bind Ms L to her object in an endless cycle of abuse and in denial of separation from the ideal object. The underlying grievance towards the mother for failing to protect her from her stepfather's intrusion is endlessly repeated and never given up.

The dream acts as a prelude to Ms L acting out at the weekend as she returns to her mother's house, despite having agreed to stay away from there. Ms L's visits home inevitably lead to arguments, which in turn result in her cutting herself. The self-harming behaviour is also used to punish the ward in a repeat of the sadomasochistic relationship with the stepfather and the mother. This pattern of behaviour is used to mask underlying anxieties about discharge and the loss of the ideal object/care offered by the unit. The self-harming behaviour expresses a grievance towards the ward for failing to protect her from the reality of discharge. In this way, Ms L tries to pull the ward staff into a sadomasochistic relationship, which undermines any healthy dependency or gratitude that she might experience towards the staff on the unit. This process defends Ms L from experiencing painful feelings of loss and gratitude by turning them into erotized feelings of grievance, which interfere with the mourning process. In the supervision group, we were able to discuss the relationship between her sadomasochistic behaviour and anxieties associated with discharge.

In the fifth clinical example, the social worker had been affected by Mrs M's apparent lack of interest in her serious and disturbing self-harming behaviour. By connecting the repetitive self-harm and attacks on her genitals with the history of childhood neglect and subsequent prostitution, the social worker was able to re-establish appropriate sympathy and concern for the patient and her neglectful attitude to herself.

Patients with borderline features are often persecuted by unreasonable and judgemental ideals that threaten their ego with accusations of inadequacy or failure leading to fragmentation and collapse. They project these ideals and subsequent feelings of blame and failure into an external object in order to protect their ego from the threats of fragmentation and collapse. However, these patients are also very attuned to the effect these hostile projections have on the recipient, as they fear the container will become overwhelmed and either retaliate or collapse. Indeed, when the recipient responds in a defensive way by counter-accusations, it can lead to bad feelings and an atmosphere of misunderstanding and blame between the patient and the recipient. This in turn may lead to a breakdown in the relationship and a fragmentation of the container. In many ways, it is true to say that these patients are looking for a "marsupial pouch" that can contain the unmanageable aspects of themselves. Patients with borderline features need to feel that people listen to them and take their difficulties seriously. However, staff who take in the patient's projections also need help in separating from the effect of these. Borderline patients need services that can provide a long-term view of their difficulties and appreciate their underlying fragility. In the first instance, the meaning of these communications needs to be digested and verbalized within the staff team. Patients with borderline features are often persecuted by harsh, judgemental self-criticism; premature interpretation of their behaviour by staff can lead to them feeling assaulted and overwhelmed (Steiner, 1993b). Teams need to consider what it is appropriate to say to patients in borderline states of mind, in what sort of clinical setting, and when to say it.

Clinical staff teams need time to reflect on their practice in shift handover and ward rounds. Psychoanalytic supervision can offer a particularly valuable perspective on patients with borderline features by making use of valuable clinical material contained within the countertransference. This form of supervision can help to counteract the tendency to think in concrete ways by helping staff to separate from the effect of the borderline patient's projections and allowing them to regain their capacity for imagination and symbolic thought; this, in turn, helps staff to think about the underlying meaning of patients' behaviour, broadening and deepening their understanding of their patients. It can also help in the assessment of clinical risk.

CHAPTER FOUR

Pinned against the ropes: psychoanalytic understanding of patients with antisocial personality disorder

This chapter focuses on the challenges involved in the treatment and care of patients with a diagnosis of psychopathic or antisocial personality disorder (APD), as it is usually referred to today. The current psychiatric diagnostic systems—ICD–10 (WHO, 1992) and DSM–5 (APA, 2013)—are primarily categorical and theoretical. A diagnosis is made by assessing the presence or absence of symptoms and behaviours. These diagnostic systems do not take any account of the individual's development or personality structure; consequently, there is no dimension for describing links between different diagnoses, and so these patients are often thought to be suffering either from paranoid schizophrenia or APD or a dual diagnosis, depending on the phase of their illness.

In this chapter, I draw upon literature in this area and suggest that this dichotomy between the psychotic and the antisocial may be too simple. If we can accept that psychotic processes may well also underlie the personality disorders, we may reach a better understanding of what takes place in the clinical setting and how staff are affected by their patients.

In his book *The Mask of Sanity*, Cleckley (1964) argues that the psychopathic character is developed to function as a defence against an underlying paranoid psychosis. He makes the point that psychopathy is not merely a "personality disorder" but is, in fact, a constructed dissimulation of a personality. Only very slowly and by a complex estimation does the conviction come upon us that we are dealing not with a complete man but with something that suggests a subtly constructed reflex machine, which can mimic the human personality perfectly. So perfect is the reproduction of a whole and normal man that anyone who examines him in a clinical setting will not be able to point out in scientific terms why or how he is not real. And yet we eventually come to know, or feel that we know, that reality—in the sense of a full, healthy experiencing of life—is not here (Cleckley, 1964).

It can be extremely difficult for mental health professionals to work with such patients if they take their explanations, rationalizations, and justifications at face value. Patients with this diagnosis often mask their disturbance behind what seems like ordinary thinking and functioning.

Hale and Dhar (2008) take up the matter of the relationship between psychopathy and psychosis in their paper "Flying a Kite—Observations on Dual (and Triple) Diagnosis". They argue that psychopathic behaviour and attitudes function as a defence against an underlying psychosis, and they describe the fluctuating presentation of patients with a diagnosis of APD as they move through different cycles of their illness. At times, patients demonstrate the characteristics of a psychopathic personality, at others they become floridly psychotic. Patients in the psychopathic stage often believe they are functioning and thinking in a normal way when, in fact, they have what Sohn (personal communication, 2005) calls "a delusion of sanity". Their thinking and behaviour is in fact highly abnormal, with envious attacks on normal functioning, often acted out through aggressive or violent acts on others' bodies or minds. In the psychotic stage, they develop a paranoid delusional system with clear psychotic symptoms.

Clinicians based in forensic or mental health settings face significant difficulties presented by patients with a diagnosis of APD. Within the clinical environment, these patients' actions often have a powerful emotional effect upon the minds of those caring for them, and these psychological states may be difficult to contain

(Ruszczynski, 2008). The forceful and concrete nature of the communications and the feelings evoked can make it challenging for clinicians to reflect on the symbolic meaning behind the patients' actions until some time after the event.

APD patients can interfere with ordinary functioning and thinking within themselves and in relation to others. For many, their extremely dysfunctional early lives and earlier disturbed relationships provide the model for future relationships. Some patients form an identification with abusive figures from their past and use violence, or threats of violence, to establish control over their objects, reversing and triumphing over traumatic situations from their childhood. Others may be extremely seductive, playing on a picture of themselves as the innocent victim of abuse or circumstances. Mental health professionals may find themselves responding to the magnetic pull of patients' unconscious as they re-enact scenarios from their history. Patients can be difficult to engage in treatment, as they often fail to see themselves as responsible for their actions or, alternatively, they normalize their behaviour (Kernberg, 2008). They are frequently secretive and deceptive in their attitude towards their care and treatment. Real capacities in themselves or others may be attacked and any development or improvement quickly undermined. Indeed, good care often provokes an envious attack or complaint against the team or the individual member of staff.

The internal world of the APD patient can be based on an idealization of the self and a pathological ego-ideal. This state of mind is maintained by establishing a model of relationships based on the need to "come out on top" at all costs. The patient gains superiority through denigration of his objects. The ego development is weak and is often based on pseudo-identifications, designed to present an impression of maturity and a capacity to learn. In fact, APD patients may suffer transient episodes of psychosis when their defences break down. Patients pick up on what is expected and adopt an identity based on the model of an ideal patient. Cartwright (2002) described this as patients' "pseudo digestive" capacities. It amounts to a form of manic reparation in which nothing is really worked through in any depth.

APD patients can form quick but superficial identifications with the object, designed to avoid difference and any acknowledgement of separation. Sohn (1985b) coined the term "identificate" to describe a process where an individual believes he is able to project himself right inside another person and take over the object's qualities via a process of intrusive projective identification. Patients internalize the qualities of the other, without any acknowledgement of their dependence upon the object or the difference between themselves and the object. Sohn makes the point that these false omnipotent structures conceal the real level of development and/or underlying illness and interfere with the possibility of treatment for the sick aspects of the self. Sohn, who has a long history of providing psychoanalytic treatment, supervision, and teaching in forensic settings, has said that APD patients lack personality, as they have failed to develop in the ordinary way. They develop defensive internal structures designed to avoid the psychic pain associated with dependence. These psychic defences function rather like an internal Mafia gang (Rosenfeld, 1971): the internal "gang" uses primitive psychological defences such as violent projective identification, mania, grandiosity, and triumph. The internal worlds of APD patients are often dominated by cruel and perverse figures that use aggressive or manic means of defending against psychic pain. There is often an idealization of the self as predator and a denigration of the other as prey (Yakeley, 2010a). This internal picture can be supported by acting out in a way that enhances the feelings of superiority and triumph over others. These patients may also use drugs and alcohol to further increase these feelings (Yakeley, 2010a).

In her paper "On Criminology", Klein (1934) describes the development of a rigid and severe superego in delinquent children. This sort of superego produces large amounts of anxiety in the ego and in the ego's relations with its objects; these individuals try to master their anxieties through the use of violent defensive mechanisms, which attack and destroy their relationship with their external objects. This creates an omnipotent world in which patients believe that they are free from anxieties associated with dependence upon the object.

Lucas (2009e) outlines the need for clinicians to tune in to the psychotic level of their patient's communication and thinking. He describes the way the psychotic part of the ego tries to murder the non-psychotic part and then tries to cover its mad deeds by denial and rationalization. Staff working with APD patients often relate how plausible, persuasive, and effective these patients are in their arguments, which frequently include the belief that their thinking is normal, they have not committed a crime, and they do not need treatment or care. Although patients may not demonstrate any obvious signs of psychopathology and may appear to be "well", there is often no sense of responsibility for their illness, their anti-social behaviour, or the events that had led to their admission. In these states of mind, staff may be seduced into colluding with patients' view of their apparent improvement and their denial of their dependence upon the mental health system to maintain their improved mental state. When working with these patients, it may be helpful to assume that a murderous attack on sanity, either within the self or within the object, is being enacted and then covered up via denial and rationalization, whether or not the patient is in the psychotic or psychopathic stage of the illness.

Staff who deal with antisocial personality say that it can take some time to recover a sense of themselves when off duty, as they are often left feeling furious, infected, or interfered with. The infectious nature of the mental states associated with APD can interfere with mental health professionals' capacity to accurately assess a patient's clinical state or level of risk. As Minne (2007) suggests in her paper on risk assessment with dangerous patients, clinicians cannot afford to forget either their patients' history or why they are being cared for in the first place. Losing touch with these clinical realities creates dangers for patients, the mental health professionals, and society at large.

Psychoanalytic supervision can provide a valuable model for working with these patients. It provides a way of thinking about patients' unconscious and psychotic levels of communication, as well as providing a model for considering the nature of the transference and countertransference relationship. This can help to support staff in their management of this patient group by adding depth to the clinical picture. It can also help staff—particularly nursing staff who are exposed to the effects of working with these patients for long periods of time—to resist the pull towards collusion enactments or thoughtless responses to patients' behaviours.

Case examples

Four case examples from supervision groups in various forensic and non-forensic mental health settings, presented over the past decade, illustrate my argument.

The psychopathic defence

A primary nurse from a treatment unit for sex offenders presented the case of Mr N.

> Mr N, in his mid-forties, had a diagnosis of APD and a history of indecent assault on minors. His index offence was a sexual assault on his girlfriend's 11-year-old daughter. The girlfriend had no knowledge of his history of paedophilia and had left her daughter in his care. Mr N said that he had not suffered any sexual or physical abuse in his childhood.

> The nurse said that Mr N could be charming and seductive on the ward, but there was always a feeling that he was "up to something". Staff suspected that he was stirring up dissatisfaction in other patients and encouraging complaints against the ward team. Mr N took a high-handed attitude towards the sex offenders' programme, claiming that he understood his condition and was no longer a threat to young girls. He believed that he had served his prison sentence and should be released. The nurse reported that despite his claims of no longer being a threat, he still referred to his child victim as his girlfriend. She did not like seeing Mr N for individual sessions, as he had a way of turning reality on its head.

> The nurse often came out of the sessions with Mr N feeling as though she had been bulldozed into seeing things from his point of view, and it took her some time to recover her own perspective. Following an individual session, Mr N made a formal complaint against her, and she discussed this subsequently in the supervision group. She said that Mr N had requested an individual session, during which he talked in the usual way

about his view that he should be discharged, as there was nothing wrong with him. The nurse pointed out the disparity between the way he referred to his victim as his girlfriend and his claim that he was cured. Mr N then became extremely abusive and shouted at her. He subsequently complained to the hospital managers that the nurse was incompetent. The nurse said she felt "like crap" after the session and had imagined taking a gun out and shooting him.

We can see how, in the index offence, Mr N gained his partner's confidence by playing the role of a serious and responsible boyfriend, and then misused this position by assaulting her daughter, interfering with his victim's enjoyment of her childhood as well as her development and future sexuality. In doing so, he also enviously attacked the mother's competence and capacity to protect her daughter.

On the unit, Mr N formed an "identificate" with an object who "knew" all he needed to know about his problems and did not need any further treatment. Indeed, he believed that he was well enough to act as an advisor to other patients on the unit. When the nurse pointed out the ongoing perversion in Mr N's thinking, confronting him with the immaturity of his boasts, he felt as though he had been assaulted. He defended himself by violently re-projecting his feelings of incompetence and inadequacy into the nurse. He then backed up these projections by making a concrete complaint in an attempt to damage her reputation. The complaint also moved attention away from questions about his level of maturity and functioning onto questions about the nurse's ability to do her work. At the same time, he enviously attacked and undermined the competence of the nurse by projecting his own immaturity and infantile state into her. This left the nurse feeling that her professionalism and maturity were being violently assaulted. The intrusiveness of this emotional assault left her feeling full of hate and wanting to shoot the patient.

Therapeutic work with APD patients involves re-introducing them to the reality of who they are and why they are being treated in a forensic or psychiatric unit (Minne, 2007). However, patients often feel assaulted when they are reminded of this reality. This reaction is particularly likely if the information is given back to the patient as a kneejerk reaction, based on the professional's wish to get something through to them or to push a psychic state that has been lodged in them back into the patient. In the case of Mr N, the nurse felt provoked and undermined by his boasts that he was able to treat himself and did not need the help of staff. Wishing to rid herself of the feeling of incompetence and to break through the grandiose and manic defence, the nurse confronted Mr N too bluntly with the reality of his on-going perversity. Although this response was understandable, it led to a repetitive argument between the patient and the nurse.

Staff need the opportunity for clinical supervision to help them think through such questions as: "What is the patient enacting?", "With what purpose?", "How could it be taken up?", and "Who needs to take it up, and with what clinical support?". The danger is that in the absence of clinical supervision, staff may feel driven to deal with patients' concrete projections by pushing them back into the patient in a premature or aggressive way, in order to protect their own sanity or sense of professionalism, thus re-enacting a sadistic countertransference. This can then lead to the patient feeling traumatized and often results in further acting out or complaints, as was the case here.

In the supervision group discussion, the nurse reflected that she had felt provoked by Mr N's behaviour. The group thought this was not surprising, given that they were starting to see it as a perverse defence designed to attack the very help and care she had to offer. In reality, Mr N was trying to destroy the nurse's authority and professionalism, pulling her into a perverse sadomasochistic relationship. However, the severity and nature of the assault meant that it was difficult for an individual member of staff not to become overwhelmed and lose her professional poise. In the supervision group, we discussed the need for two members of staff to work as his primary nurses. In future, the two nurses would see Mr N together, which would allow them to work as a team and reduce the likelihood of any one individual being overwhelmed by his perverse and provocative thinking and behaviour. I suggested that the team should explain that this approach was required by the nature of Mr N's clinical condition. We also agreed to meet to discuss the case in supervision on a regular and on-going basis.

Delinquent defence

A primary nurse from an acute psychiatric ward presented the case of Mr O.

Mr O, a patient in his late forties, had been transferred from prison as part of the court diversion programme six months previously. He had a history of getting drunk and starting fights. Following a fight outside a pub in which he stabbed another man in the ear, resulting in the victim's hearing loss, Mr O was convicted of grievous bodily harm. He maintained that the stabbing was an act of self-defence, but while in prison he complained of hearing voices and was diagnosed with paranoid schizophrenia and transferred to an acute psychiatric ward. Mr O lived with his mother but forbade staff from talking to her, claiming that she was controlling and manipulative. The nurse mentioned in passing that his mother had once told Social Services that Mr O bullied and physically attacked her. He had not worked for many years but spent his time drinking in a local pub and would get into fights from time to time. Mr O's father was described as having been rather weak and ineffectual; he had died during Mr O's teens.

The nurse working with Mr O told the supervision group that Mr O had stopped participating in the therapeutic programme for some time, arguing that he did not like the groups. He had developed a routine of sleeping until late morning, having lunch, then leaving the ward and returning several hours later, smelling of drink. The occupational therapist said that on one occasion Mr O had attended an art group and had painted a miniature figure. When asked to say something about it, he described it as a black man who was about to be electrocuted on death row. The nurse said that Mr O heard mocking voices saying that he was a "useless shit".

The ward manager stated that the nursing team felt completely stuck, as every time they gave Mr O a discharge date, he would tell the psychiatric registrar that he was suicidal. She believed that he played up his symptoms to the psychiatric registrar on the ward and in front of the consultant in the Care Programme

Approach (CPA) meetings, resulting in the consultant agreeing to postpone his discharge. Another nurse added that he had seen Mr O laughing with another patient in the day room directly after his CPA. The ward manager said the nursing team were frustrated, as they did not feel Mr O should still be on the ward, believing that he was not genuinely suicidal or benefiting from his admission. She said that she felt the medical team were ignoring the nursing team's opinion. Mr O became abusive and hostile when the nurse pointed out that he was undermining his treatment programme by leaving the ward every afternoon and "treating the ward like a hotel". Mr O responded by becoming verbally aggressive and intimidating and subsequently took out a complaint against the nurse, claiming she was unprofessional in her manner.

Mr O used the diagnosis of mental illness to manipulate his situation, causing a split between the nursing and medical teams. He maintained a view of himself as an ill man who could take no responsibility for himself or his difficulties, while at the same time believing that he should be free to go to the pub. Mr O acted as if his behaviour were perfectly acceptable, and the nurse was made to feel as if she had acted in a tyrannical way by questioning his ritual visits to the pub. In this way, Mr O denied both his dependence on drink and the link between his drinking and his violence. Mr O did not question the fact that his pattern of behaviour and drinking increased his risk of violence and reoffending but, rather, on the contrary, acted as though this was part of a therapeutic pattern to be maintained at all costs. Mr O became aggressive and intimidating when the nurse questioned his attitude towards treatment, as this interfered with his belief that he was a hotel guest going out for a harmless lunchtime drink.

Mr O functioned like a tyrannical infant who believed that he should be looked after, without any expectation of development or change. He did not acknowledge any gratitude or debt towards the people he depended on, but acted as though he should be cared for cost-free. He projected his sane awareness of his infantile state into the voice that called him a "useless shit" and then treated this voice as if it was a mad, victimizing part of his mind that was making bizarre and savage accusations without justification. The reality was that this critical voice represented the sane part of Mr O's mind, because it disapproved of his delinquent and irresponsible behaviour. The underlying paranoid state broke through when the nurse challenged his delinquent attitude towards his illness. He then projected the psychosis into the nurse by complaining that she behaved in a tyrannical and judgemental way. In doing so, he denied the significance of his admission to the ward and the need for treatment of his delinquency and underlying paranoid personality structure.

Mr O had a delinquent relationship with care, which he felt was his entitlement and may have represented a repetition of an abusive relationship with his mother. However, although this was an important part of the clinical picture, it failed to acknowledge the problem of the underlying feeling of inadequacy and humiliation when he was made to feel small. This was mainly denied through the delinquent defence but broke through when the patient consumed alcohol or was asked to examine his behaviour. The nursing and medical teams were split in picking up two different levels of the patient's presentation. The nursing staff were aware of the delinquent attitude towards treatment but were not in tune with the patient's underlying feeling of humiliation and inadequacy. The medical team were not in tune with the delinquency but did pick up on the patient's underlying immaturity and suicidal state. The split between the two teams did not allow both aspects of the clinical picture to come together. Discussion in the supervision group allowed the multidisciplinary team to reduce the split in their thinking and consider different elements of the presentation. As a consequence a management plan was put in place, which required Mr O to attend his occupational and therapeutic programme. When he failed to attend his programme, his nurse would arrange a meeting to discuss his avoidance of treatment and how this meant he was not taking his underlying difficulties or his risk factors seriously.

Patients are often extremely sensitive to existing splits in the multidisciplinary team, and some patients are able to exacerbate these splits. This form of splitting aims to stop the clinical team gathering impressions together. If this sort of splitting goes on unchecked, it can undermine the capacity of the clinical team to think effectively about the patient and interferes with appropriate clinical management. Supervision can be used to understand the function of the splitting process as well as provide a space where different professional disciplines and/or individuals can examine the different ways they may have been caught up in it. This process can then restore good relationships between professionals and disciplines.

The delusional defence

A ward manager from a medium-secure unit presented the case of Mr P.

Mr P, a married man in his forties, had attacked his pregnant wife, causing her to miscarry. He was admitted to the unit quite soon after the assault, in an agitated and manic state, complaining that a secret religious sect was planning to replace Allah with an evil impostor. He believed that the evil impostor had taken the form of his unborn child, whom he had attacked in an attempt to defend his religion.

Mr P had had a successful academic career before working in his father's property development business, in which he was eventually made a partner. Two years later, he left his father's business and started a rival firm. Several years after that, he bought his father's old company in an aggressive takeover bid. At around the same time, Mr P's wife announced that she was pregnant with their first child. His wife reported that several days before the assault he had started to become rather agitated and low in mood. Mr P's manic and agitated presentation on admission soon calmed down after he had been given anti-psychotic medication, and he began to engage with the therapeutic programme. After a few weeks, he settled into the role of a model patient and started to offer advice and counsel to other patients in the unit. The ward manager said that the forensic psychiatrist leading the team had developed a view that Mr P had been the victim of a transient psychotic illness that had been successfully treated by medication, which was a view that Mr P was keen to support and adopt. The ward manager felt that Mr P was being rushed towards discharge in an unusual way, as if he occupied the position of a "special patient", and that Mr P's cold indifference to his index offence and lack of remorse "sent shivers down his spine".

Mr P presented a picture of himself as a model son, while he was actually plotting his father's downfall. The aggressive and manic acquisition of his father's company began to cause financial difficulties for the company and psychological difficulties for Mr P's psyche, and these factors precipitated his breakdown. Mr P's progress was based on his ability to play the part of a devoted son and employee while planning an aggressive takeover at the same time. There was no acknowledgement of any need for help or gratitude for what others had done for him. He began to suffer from a depressive breakdown as his manic and grandiose mental state began to collapse. He began to feel persecuted by the emergence of the sane part of his mind, which brought to his attention the damaging nature of his psychopathic defence. The sane part of his mind, which threatened to cause a complete depressive breakdown, was then projected into his unborn child. In his paranoid delusional system, the child became the destructive force that threatened to undermine Allah, the father. As the threat of the depressive breakdown increased, his paranoid defence against the breakdown also increased, and the attack on the unborn child represented a concrete psychotic attempt to get rid of the sane part of his mind.

The acute stages of Mr P's psychosis quickly settled down after his admission to the ward and treatment with anti-psychotic medication. Quite soon after his admission and recovery from the acute stages of his illness, he adopted a "medical explanation" for the episode, believing he had suffered a brief psychotic illness, which was now resolved with treatment.

The ward manager's countertransference to Mr P's cold indifference drew attention to an underlying problem. His rivalrous relationship with his father was re-enacted on the ward, as he fraudulently played the role of the model patient while subtly taking over the staff's therapeutic function, projecting his difficulties into the other patients in the unit while avoiding any real examination of his own problems. The idea that Mr P had suffered from a transient psychotic episode was seized and used to explain away his actions, as if the index offence had nothing to do with him and did not need further exploration or understanding. In this way, Mr P and certain elements of the clinical team minimized the connection between Mr P's index offence and his psychopathic behaviour in relation to his father's business. It also distanced Mr P from any feeling of guilt or responsibility for his actions, his illness, or his risk factors. The ward manager's countertransference indicated that their psychiatric authority was being duped, undermined by the patient's intelligence and ability to play the role of the dutiful patient.

Repetition of the index offence on the inpatient unit

A keyworker from a sex offenders' treatment programme presented the case of Mr Q.

> Mr Q was a middle-aged man with a 20-year history of offences ranging from fraud to rape. The current index offence involved Mr Q standing by his front door with a white stick in his hand and asking a woman passing by to help him with something in his flat. Once inside, Mr Q had pulled out a gun, trapping the woman in the corner of a room, where he raped her.
>
> Mr Q's father was a drug dealer who had frequently attacked Mr Q's mother and had left the family home when Mr Q was very young. His childhood was described as disruptive, and he was expelled from several schools as a result of truanting and disturbing behaviour in the classroom. He was convicted of various offences during his teens, including fraud and anti-social behaviour.
>
> Mr Q had a diagnosis of APD with borderline traits. The keyworker described him as an extremely intimidating and unpleasant man, who was uncooperative and hostile to staff and patients alike. Mr Q tended to hijack the therapeutic groups for his own agenda and would launch into speeches about his belief that he was being held illegally, because there was nothing

wrong with him. At times, other patients became so fed up with Mr Q's behaviour that they threatened to attack him, and he had to be put into seclusion for his own safety. The keyworker said that Mr Q had a history of taking out complaints against members of staff who questioned him, and he often demanded to see the consultant of the unit or senior hospital manager to discuss his grievances. These meetings increased his sense of self-importance, as he saw himself as someone with friends in high places, who boasted that he could have staff removed from the ward if they did not comply with his wishes.

The keyworker reported that Mr Q had a history of "grooming" newly qualified female staff. In the previous week, Mr Q had approached a nurse who was not part of his primary care team, claiming that he felt like harming himself, and he engaged her in a prolonged discussion. When the keyworker found the couple talking in a quiet corner of the unit, he immediately felt guilty and responsible, fearing that he had failed to protect his colleague from his patient. When he asked what was going on, the newly qualified member of staff said that Mr Q was in a distressed state, and she was counselling him. When he questioned why Mr Q had not asked to see him, as his keyworker, the patient claimed that he should be free to talk to whomever he wanted and that he did not find the keyworker helpful. Mr Q went straight to the ward manager and demanded to be given a new keyworker. When his request was denied, he became extremely abusive, claiming that this breached his human rights. He said he was going to have the keyworker and the ward manager removed from the unit, and yet again demanded to have a meeting with the consultant. The keyworker finished the presentation by saying that he was fed up with the patient's complaints, because his professional status and capacity to do his work was constantly undermined. Mr Q made him feel completely useless; he often went home in a restless, miserable state of mind, and things had deteriorated so much that he was having nightmares about the patient.

In his index offence, Mr Q impersonated a man in need of help in order to trap his victim. By overpowering and raping his victim, he enhanced his feeling of potency and control over the victim. He took what he wanted, aggressively, violently, and without any thought for the woman's wishes or desires. Mr Q symbolically repeated the index offence on the unit by fraudulently playing the role of a man in need of help and trapping the young female member of staff in a corner with threats of self-harm. He aggressively stole therapeutic contact that did not belong to him, aware of his care plan, which specified that he was only offered individual time by members of his primary team. He replicated the same aggressive, fraudulent behaviour displayed in the index offence on the ward, interfering with normal convention by taking what he wanted without consent. In this way, he may have identified with his father's intoxicated and violent way of operating, taking what he wanted from a woman with no concern for her. Fuel was added to Mr Q's manic and grandiose state of mind when he was granted a meeting with the consultant to voice his complaints, believing he had been successful in splitting the medical consultant from the keyworker. The keyworker's countertransference on finding the newly qualified nurse talking to the patient highlights the destructive nature of Mr Q's relationship with care and help. The keyworker felt that he had been unable to protect the newly qualified member of staff from an abusive and corrupting experience. This gave an indication of the way in which Mr Q maintained his psychic retreat as he violently perverted and attacked offers of help, thus triumphing over his difficulties and need for help. The keyworker's countertransference related to his fear that Mr Q used pseudo-vulnerability in order to elicit help from vulnerable individuals. Then, in a repetition of the index offence, he trapped the victim and forcibly took something that did not belong to him.

Discussion

Patients with a diagnosis of APD present their carers with challenging clinical problems. Their tendency towards violent actions can also be seductive and charming, playing carers off against one another. New staff are particularly vulnerable, as patients may seduce them into believing that they can be "rescued" or that they have a special relationship.

The threat posed by some of these patients is not just confined to their physical violence; it also relates to the psychological effect they can have on those caring for them. There can be a perverse attitude towards care that is carried over into their relationships with mental health professionals, and their attack on good care, combined with their envy of those caring for them, can undermine the environment necessary for good therapeutic work. They may also form an identificate in which they take in and take over the attributes of others in an attempt to provide the personality with some sense of meaning and coherence. This is the basis of a false identity that conceals the patient's underlying difficulties and need for treatment.

APD patients use psychotic mechanisms to defend themselves against depressive and/or persecutory anxieties, and for some patients the antisocial character structure functions as a defence against an underlying paranoid psychosis. It may be more accurate to think of these patients as suffering from a dual diagnosis. This involves two distinct psychic structures represented by the different clinical presentations. The underlying psychic structures operate in a dynamic relationship within the patient's personality. This dynamic relationship responds to external and internal pressures as the balance of influence alternates between one set of psychic defences and psychic organization and another (Hale & Dhar, 2008).

Clinical supervision and opportunities for reflective practice are essential for good psychological care of such patients and the staff involved with them. Thinking about the internal world of the patient, the unconscious communication, and the transference–countertransference and providing a model for thinking about different levels of the mind are particularly important when dealing with antisocial patients, as clinicians may need to tune in to the psychotic processes of patients' actions and behaviours (see chapter 2). Psychoanalytic supervision, by focusing on the quality of the therapeutic engagement, can add an essential dimension to risk assessment and suitability for treatment (Yakeley, 2010b). Accurate risk assessment requires a dynamic model of the patient's mind that takes account of the relationships between different aspects of the patient's internal world. Risk assessment also needs to take account of the way the patient's mental state influences changes in the level of risk.

It is vital that managers understand the complex nature of APD, in order to support frontline staff and to be familiar with the clinical problems presented by these patients. Clinical supervision and consultation is a necessity for the psychological well-being of staff and patients alike. These patients require a team approach, and team processes also need to be addressed and understood in supervision. At times, it may be appropriate to look at a patient's complaint as a communication about an underlying clinical problem. It is hoped that this might help to reduce breaches in boundaries or acting out by both staff and patients.

In the first case study, the supervision group was able to think about the way Mr N defended himself from the reality of his immature and perverse mental state by projecting his incompetence into other patients on the programme. This left him free to maintain a belief that he was cured of his problems, and he forced the primary nurse to listen to his propaganda. When the nurse challenged his belief that he was cured and reminded him of his perversion, he felt assaulted and made a complaint. The supervisor then proposed a plan to offer on-going supervision and support for the nurse in order to think through her interactions with the patient. In this instance, the provocative aggressive and perverse nature of the patient provoked the nurse into arguments with Mr N. The nurse needed help with containing her understandably strong countertransferential reactions to his provocations. The supervision group gave the nurse a place where she could discuss and think about the feelings of frustration in order to restore and maintain professional poise.

In the second case study, the supervisor made use of the primary nurse's countertransference to understand the split between the nursing and medical view. Although Mr O maintained an irresponsible attitude towards treatment, he also used his delinquency to conceal an underlying paranoia and feelings of inadequacy and humiliation. The supervision group was able to help the team integrate the nursing and medical view and regain its clinical focus.

With the third case study, the supervisor made use of the ward manager's countertransference in conjunction with thoughts about Mr P's history and his clinical presentation on the ward to draw a dynamic formulation. The team were then able to reflect on the fact that he was acting out on the ward his previous psychopathology with his rivalrous takeover of the staff team's function in relation to himself and other patients.

The fourth case study drew attention to the repetition of Mr Q's index offence on the ward, and this raised questions around his availability for treatment. When the keyworker stepped in to protect the inexperienced member of staff from a symbolic repetition of the index offence, the patient retaliated by trying to spoil and tarnish the keyworker's reputation. The supervisor also pointed out the way the patient was able to split the consultant psychiatrist from his nursing colleagues by creating collusion with the patient's manic and perverse defence. The nurse's countertransferential feeling that he had not been able to protect the new nurse from exploitation was a constant clinical problem in Mr Q's treatment.

APD patients communicate their underlying disturbance through powerful psychological mechanisms and concrete physical actions as they rid themselves of unwanted aspects of their internal worlds. Patients may act in a way intended to produce a specific reaction in their carers, prompting mental health professionals to respond in line with a "script" provided for them. These patients have a complicated relationship with care and may attack and undermine the therapeutic team's efforts. They may also have a malignant relationship with authority, and they tend to identify with bullying and controlling figures. At times, the strength of feelings evoked can leave staff feeling as if they are "pinned against the ropes", and professionals may either act out in response to patients' provocations or distance themselves for fear of acting out. Therapeutic work is beset with dangers and difficulties, and patients may only reveal their true interest in therapy over time. Antisocial patients can also conceal the real nature of their difficulties, and re-enactments of the index offence in ward settings may be subtle and repetitive.

In these difficult circumstances, clinical supervision and opportunities for reflective practice provide an essential support for staff. As Minne states, psychoanalytic understanding can provide "a model for thinking about the contagious effects of anti-social personality disordered patients" (Minne, 2008, p. 28). Antisocial patients may use therapeutic relationships in corrupt ways that avoid meaningful engagement. Psychoanalytic supervision then provides staff with an opportunity to reflect on the destructive nature of such relationships and the meaning of the patient's confusing behaviour. Understanding the countertransference with such patients is essential in helping to decontaminate unhealthy aspects of the clinical situation that get lodged inside staff in an unhelpful way. Antisocial patients often project feelings of guilt and a sense of responsibility. They may also seek corrupt relationships and induce staff into sadomasochistic relationships. The supervisor is in the privileged position of remaining less contaminated and at a distance from the direct effects of the patient's communications and is more free to think about the unconscious meaning of the actions and reactions, thus turning the dyad of mental health professional and patient, action and reaction, into a triadic relationship, with the supervisor or supervision group representing thought and meaning.

CHAPTER FIVE

Tuning in
to the psychotic wavelength

Patients in psychotic states of mind often communicate their psychological problems through "concrete thinking" or "concrete actions". This form of thinking is rigid and lacks the "as-if" quality necessary for symbolic thought; consequently, there is no room for associations or imagination. This sort of communication is stripped of its psychological meaning and does not convey emotional significance in an accessible way, exemplified in the distinction drawn by Hanna Segal (1957) between the "symbol", which is used to represent things and conveys emotional significance, and the "symbolic equation", which is felt to be the thing in itself (see chapter 1).

The literal and concrete nature of the communication does not invite the listener to freely associate to the content but, rather, invites a literal and concrete response. Consequently, mental health professionals working with psychotic patients have the job of trying to put some emotional meaning and life back into a lifeless communication by using their own capacity for symbolic thought, free association, and imagination. Richard Lucas described this level of communication as the "psychotic wavelength" and argued that staff need to "tune in" to this psychotic wavelength (Lucas,

2009e). When staff are able to "tune in" to their patients' communications in this way, it can help to change patients' monologue about their delusional world into a meaningful dialogue about their psychic state.

However, the deadening effect of the concrete communication can interfere with mental health professionals' ordinary capacity to think about their patients. Reflective practice and supervision groups help staff to recover their capacity to relate to their patients in an emotionally meaningful way. This should be seen not as an unnecessary luxury but, rather, as an essential part of all good mental health practice. I have found that a psychoanalytic approach is particularly valuable when trying to understand psychotic states of mind. This is not to say that it is the only way of thinking about psychotic states; more that it can complement other ways of thinking by shining a light on unconscious psychological processes. Although it can be argued that psychoanalytic psychotherapy may be of limited benefit for patients suffering from schizophrenia, psychoanalytic ideas provide an invaluable insight into the psychotic mind and psychotic means of communication. These insights, by helping staff with clinical understanding and management, can, in turn, assist them in their assessment of patients' needs in order to provide the right sort of psychological, medical, and social support.

Case examples

Understanding the patient's concrete communication through the countertransference

A primary nurse, a ward manager, and an occupational therapist from an inpatient unit presented the case of Ms R.

Ms R, 32 years old and with a diagnosis of schizophrenia, had been causing many problems on the ward. According to the primary nurse, the patient presented in a child-like way and had a habit of taking all of her clothes off. The ward manager added that the other patients found this sort of behaviour upsetting, and the nursing staff were becoming exasperated. The ward manager said that there had been no change in the patient's behaviour since her admission. The occupational therapist added that Ms R was acting in such an immature way that she had to be removed from ward activities. I asked the team to tell me something of the patient's history and family circumstances. The primary nurse said that the patient lived at home with her parents and spent long periods of time on her own, alone in her bedroom. She had shown very little capacity to stick to any education since her late teens or to hold down a job. However, her father still believed that she was capable of getting a job and getting married. The ward manager said that the father was a dominant character who believed that his daughter should "pull herself together and find a husband and a job". The primary nurse added that the patient expressed a delusional belief that "a large man is sitting on top of my head", and that this was reported by Ms R in a flat, lifeless way, devoid of any emotion.

The literal and concrete nature of Ms R's communication that "a large man is sitting on top of my head" did not invite, or leave room for, associations. The listener was invited either to agree with the patient and join a meaningless delusional monologue about the man on the patient's head, or to disagree, say that there is no man on her head, and get into an equally meaningless argument. The flattened affect and literal statement of concrete fact, "a large man is sitting on top of my head", does not invite any engagement with the listener on the symbolic level, because the statement seems to be designed to keep out the possibility of symbolic meaning and emotional connection. Not surprisingly, mental health professionals can respond to these deadened psychotic monologues either by arguing or by ignoring them.

My interpretation was that the man sitting on Ms R's head was her father, who was crushing her with his expectations of normal development, which she did not feel able to meet. She experienced her father as trying to force her into a marriage or a job because of his own preoccupations and anxieties. This situation was re-enacted on the ward as the staff team were trying to push the patient to progress with her treatment before really understanding her underlying difficulties. Ms R was protesting against these expectations by stripping off and demanding that people look at her. The problem was that she presented her problem through concrete action that demanded attention to her body rather than to her mind.

Ms R's behaviour gave an accurate picture of her emotional age: her behaviour was more appropriate to a 3-year-old girl than to a 32-year-old woman. I suggested to the primary nurse and the nursing team that they convey to Ms R that they understood her need for someone to see her and take her seriously. The primary nurse needed to help Ms R to explore her anxieties about being forced into a job or marriage, and to explain that she understood that Ms R felt under pressure to fit in with the ward's demands for progress, as with her parents' expectations. I also suggested that the primary nurse might helpfully explore the patient's feelings about her life and what her aspirations were. At the same time, we discussed the need for the nursing staff to encourage Ms R to attend her occupational therapy programme. If Ms R started to strip off her clothes, they might say that they understood that it must be difficult for her to behave in an ordinary way when she felt crushed by demands and expectations. I also suggested that they convey how difficult it must be for Ms R to think about herself and what she wanted from life when she was being told what to do by the man who sat on her head. The staff could then say that they thought Ms R was trying to get them to look at her body, but that they also needed to think with her about her thoughts and feelings.

The following week, the team presented Ms R again, saying that there had been a marked improvement both in her behaviour and in her mental state. The ward manager explained that they had instigated a care plan, which the team now followed. When Ms R started to strip off her clothes, staff would take her to her room and explain that they understood she was anxious about things and that she would have an opportunity to talk to her primary nurse and psychologist about her anxieties. The occupational therapist added that Ms R had started to attend occupational therapy on a more regular basis and seemed more able to concentrate. We talked about the need for the ward to instigate some work with the family to help them think about Ms R in a more realistic way, which would include some acknowledgement of her problems.

Two weeks later, the ward manager said that they had met with the family. This time, with some encouragement from the primary nurse, Ms R's mother had found her voice. She had complained that the father had unrealistic expectations of their daughter and that they had to become more realistic. The primary nurse said that Ms R's mental state improved considerably after this meeting. We discussed the need for a discharge plan to support the patient following discharge. It was agreed that she would need the one-to-one work to continue, as well as referral to a day hospital where they might continue the rehabilitation programme and family work. Several weeks later, Ms R was discharged back to her family with a referral to the community psychiatric team for medication and individual and family work. The ward team felt good about the work that had been done with Ms R and pleased with the way the team had worked together.

A month or so later, the ward manager started the supervision group by saying that there was something that the group urgently needed to discuss. Ms R had been readmitted to the ward after taking an overdose in an agitated state. The ward manager said that Ms R had regressed to her old behaviour but was more rebellious than she had been on previous admissions. She was shouting at staff and demanding that they make her cups of tea and tidy her room. The ward manager said, with some feeling, that something urgently needed to be done, as she was sure Ms R would be assaulted by one of the other patients if her provocative behaviour continued. The primary nurse went on to say that the community psychiatric team had discharged Ms R, and her father had insisted that she join a dating agency and sign on at the Job Centre. The feeling in the staff team was that we had to come up with an urgent solution to the clinical problem, or else there would be some sort of explosive incident.

My thoughts were that this was communicating something about the patient's internal world through a split countertransference. On the one hand, the staff team felt that they were being driven mad by Ms R's tyrannical and bullying behaviour, while, on the other, they were concerned that her immature and reckless behaviour would lead to some sort of assault on her person from other patients. Through her behaviour, the staff were given an experience of what it was like to be Ms R. She felt tyrannized by her father's demands that she should fit in with his wishes, while at the same time she demonstrated that she was a rebellious child who was not going to behave as expected. I said that I thought the staff could be firm but sympathetic by saying to Ms R that they understood that she felt bossed around and pressured into doing what the man on her head wanted, and that she felt there was no room for her to decide what she wanted or what she was looking for. I also thought it was important for the team to acknowledge that Ms R was probably right in thinking that she was not ready to stand up to other people's demands and expectations and would need ongoing occupational, social, and psychological support. We discussed the requirement for the ward team to reassess Ms R's discharge plan, including her living arrangements. This should include an assessment of community services, either by visiting them or by inviting them in to ward rounds. The inpatient unit needed to get a picture from the community team regarding the type of support available and the length of time they would be able to offer Ms R that support. In this way, they could match up what they thought the patient needed post-discharge with what was actually available.

Mental health professionals—especially nursing staff who are with patients for long periods of time and see patients in different roles—need time in handovers, reflective practice, and supervision to recover their feelings along with their capacity to use their imagination or capacity to free-associate. Supervisors are in a privileged position: not working directly with the patient and thus not being affected by the patients' concrete projections, they can encourage and enable staff to separate themselves from the effects of the patients' projections while using their imagination to think about the meaning of the communications. So, for example, the nurse or staff group may begin to think that the delusional image of the large man sitting on her head is actually related to Ms R's feeling weighed down and crushed by her father's expectations. Indeed, Ms R had "the weight of the world on her shoulders". Thus, we can put the missing emotional significance back into the concrete communication. This hypothesis then needs to be critically examined and thought about in relation to other pieces of information from the clinical picture to see if it makes any sense.

This sort of information can complement observations about the patient's behaviour and give access to the patient's internal world. It can also add depth and complexity to the understanding of the patient's mental state and symptomatology. It provides us with a way of turning Ms R's delusional monologue about the man on her head into a dialogue about her feelings. This means that we shift the ground from a discussion about the nature of physical reality to a discussion about the nature of her emotional reality. When this happens, staff are able to tune in to the part of the patient that is searching for someone who can convert the concrete physical communication into an emotionally meaningful dialogue.

Helping staff to separate from the effects of the patient's rationalization

A CPN said that he would like to talk about a new case, as he did not know what to make of it.

> Mr S, 45 years old, with a diagnosis of paranoid schizophrenia, had been living in a mental health hostel for a number of years. The previous week, the CPN had received a phone call from the hostel manager, saying that Mr S was becoming increasingly isolated and argumentative with other residents. The CPN said that he arranged to visit Mr S during the subsequent week and, following that meeting, met with the hostel manager.

> The CPN reported that Mr S came across as a calm and rational man who said that the other residents were tapping on the pipes and trying to drive him mad. This was making him feel worse, and, consequently, he wanted to move into his own flat. I asked the CPN to tell us his assessment of the patient's mental state. He said that he did not feel that there were any signs or symptoms of psychosis and that Mr S was able to hold a rational conversation about the difficulties he had been having in the hostel. The CPN said that he was left wondering whether the

other residents were actually tapping on the pipes. He went on to say that he had spoken to the housing association about the possibility of obtaining a single flat for Mr S. The CPN had then spoken to the manager of the hostel, who confirmed that Mr S had been behaving in a bizarre way and losing his temper with other residents. The hostel manager also said that Mr S had been refusing to take his anti-psychotic medication for several weeks, as he did not believe he had a mental illness.

I asked the CPN if he could identify what he felt while he was with Mr S. He said that he felt that Mr S was very intense, guarded, and a bit fixed in his views, but he wondered whether this was to do with the fact that he was a relatively new CPN. I then asked him whether he knew anything about Mr S's delusional beliefs. He said that he did not, but he did remember seeing a description in the notes of Mr S's delusional beliefs from a previous admission two years previously. Mr S had been detained under mental health legislation in a paranoid state, saying that he had bought some drugs from the IRA in the 1980s and they had been pursuing him for the money ever since.

I thought that Mr S was breaking down but his psychosis was being concealed by his rationalization. I suggested that the CPN go back to see Mr S and ask him why he thought the other residents were banging on the pipes. In relation to the flat, I thought that he might ask Mr S why he believed that moving to a single flat was the answer to his problems. Lastly, I thought it would be helpful if the CPN recorded his thoughts and feelings about what Mr S was saying immediately following their meetings.

The following week, the CPN came to the supervision group and said that he had been to see the hostel manager, who reported that Mr S's behaviour was getting worse and they might have to consider asking him to leave. He then went on to describe his meeting with Mr S. He said that the patient started quite calmly, talking in a measured way, but became increasingly intense and angry. When Mr S started to talk about the other residents tapping on the pipes, the CPN asked him why he thought they were doing this. Mr S became a little more agitated and said that the other residents were all connected with the IRA and were trying to drive him mad. At this point the CPN told the supervision group that he had decided to "spell out" the reality to Mr S. He informed Mr S that the hostel manager reported that Mr S was becoming aggressive to other residents, not the other way around. Suddenly Mr S became very angry, saying that he could not believe that the CPN was accusing him of lying. The CPN told the group that he felt slightly intimidated by Mr S and rather taken aback by the strength of Mr S's feelings. After a pause in his presentation, the CPN added that Mr S's room was getting messier and that he seemed to have stopped washing.

In the supervision group, we were able to think about Mr S and his difficulties by using Bion's model, in which he described a split in the patient's ego between the psychotic and non-psychotic part of the personality (Bion, 1957). The psychotic part of the personality then hates all emotional links and ties, fragments any capacity to perceive or register emotional difficulties or conflicts, operates in an omnipotent way, and hates the recognition of dependence upon others for help. The psychotic part also tries to solve complex emotional problems through concrete physical actions. The psychotic part of the personality is in deadly rivalry with the non-psychotic or sane part of the personality, which does register emotions and emotional problems and is able to recognize dependence on others for help.

From our discussions, the group decided that Mr S was dominated by the psychotic part of his mind that had drugged him in order to defend himself against the perception of reality. The reality was that Mr S was a man with a psychotic illness, living in a hostel for people with serious and long-standing psychiatric illnesses. However, the psychotic part of Mr S denied this reality by presenting himself to himself as a calm, reasonable man, surrounded by tyrannical people who were trying to drive him mad.

The psychotic part of Mr S's personality projected his sane but disturbing insight—that he was a man suffering from a mental illness—onto the other residents. This disturbing realization always threatened to push itself back into Mr S's mind and undermine his belief that there was nothing wrong with him. The evacuation of Mr S's sanity left a space, which he filled with a delusional system in which he maintained a psychotic belief that he was the sane one, and his only problem was that he needed to move away physically from the other residents. Indeed, he believed that his sanity depended upon his ability to get away from these residents, who were trying to drive him mad. In this way, Mr S turned reality on its head: dominated by a tyrannical psychotic belief that he did not have any problems and did not need any help, he treated his sanity as if it were the enemy threatening to cause a breakdown. In his delusional system, the terrorist IRA represented Mr S's sanity, and his psychosis was represented by his calm "no-problem" presentation. The psychotic part of Mr S then rationalized his version of reality by trying to recruit the CPN into his psychosis, by getting him to agree that he was perfectly sane and reasonable in his request to move out of the mental health hostel, as if getting away from the hostel would get him away from his insanity, thus solving his problems—whereas, on the contrary, in that case Mr S would be moved further away from the recognition that he was a man with a psychiatric illness who needed the support and help of a CMHT and a mental health hostel; he would move further into a self-created delusional world in which there was no acknowledgement of any problems and no need for any help. His psychotic part feared that insight would destroy his omnipotent belief in his independence and his way of dealing with emotional problems, which was to distance himself from them. However, the calm, psychotic state broke down when the CPN said that he had spoken to the hostel manager, who had contradicted Mr S's version of events.

In a paper describing his approach to the treatment of psychotic patients, Bion outlined the need for mental health professionals to address themselves to the sane part of the patient (Bion, 1955, p. 225). When this is not available, staff need to identify and address a sane member of the family or person within the patient's social circle. In many ways, the hostel manager was the sane one in Mr S's social structure, and she needed to be supported in her difficult role with Mr S. I said to the CPN that he needed to reassure the hostel manager that he was taking her concerns seriously and that she would be invited to an urgent review of Mr S's care. I also thought that the CPN needed to have an urgent discussion with Mr S's consultant psychiatrist about his mental state and threatening behaviour and also his cessation of medication.

The CPN asked me how he and the consultant might go about

talking to Mr S, as he did not want to provoke an aggressive out-
burst. The CPN needed to discuss the risks factors with the consultant and CMHT leader. I suggested that they might start by saying
to Mr S that they understood it must be quite difficult for him to be
dominated by a part of himself that believed he could deal with any
emotional problem by distancing himself or moving away from the
mental health hostel. I also thought they might say to him that it
must be difficult being told what to do by a part of himself that
refused to acknowledge his need for help and support. If he failed
to engage with this discussion, they could remind him that he had
a history of relapsing when discharged from psychiatric care, and
that they strongly recommend he start taking his medication again,
as it would help him to manage his feelings about needing to be
self-sufficient and would, hopefully, enable him to re-engage with
the care team.

Two weeks later, the CPN said that he and the consultant had
met with Mr S, and they had taken up some of the things
I suggested in the previous supervision session. The CPN
said that although Mr S started by arguing, he quickly settled
down when he realized that both his CPN and the consultant were serious in their concerns. The CPN said that he was
surprised Mr S had listened and felt that he seemed to be
relieved. The CPN said that he had an agreement with the
hostel manager that he would visit every fortnight, and they
would invite her to Mr S's CPA meeting on a regular basis.
Several weeks later, the CPN reported that Mr S was taking a
small dose of anti-psychotic medication. This seemed to help
him to settle down, and he had even started to engage with
the other residents.

Helping mental health professionals to separate themselves
from an urge to rescue the patient

A psychiatrist attached to an inpatient service presented the case
of Mr T.

Mr T was a 30-year-old man with a diagnosis of paranoid
schizophrenia, and the psychiatrist had been asked to assess

him in prison as part of the court diversion scheme. Mr T had been arrested and charged with breaking and entering and threatening behaviour. He had broken into a woman's house, taken off his clothes, and demanded sex. When the woman refused, he just stood there, saying that she must have sex with him. Mr T did not harm the woman concerned but continued to demand sex. The woman phoned the police, and the man was arrested and charged.

The psychiatrist told the supervision group that she had assessed Mr T and found him to be pleasant and unthreatening. He had been very passive, sitting and looking at her with wide eyes and a pleasant smile. Mr T had been bullied at school but then started fighting and was eventually expelled. He started smoking marijuana during his teens and was arrested several times for stealing. He had his first psychotic breakdown when he was 18 years old, and he developed a delusion that he was Christ. He had been in and out of forensic hostels, prison, and inpatient mental health units ever since.

The psychiatrist wanted to suggest to the magistrate that Mr T should be admitted to the acute admission ward to which she was attached. However, the psychiatrist's colleagues were not very happy about admitting him to the ward, because they did not think that they would be able to contain him and thought they would have difficulty placing him in a rehabilitation hostel because of his antisocial behaviour.

The psychiatrist told the supervision group that she did not think Mr T should be sent to prison, as he was psychiatrically ill. She was upset that no one seemed to want him and said that services were repeating the history of his past by passing him from "pillar to post". She went on to say, with some feeling, that she thought he needed a period of stability and treatment. In the discussion, it became apparent that the psychiatrist had become quite attached to and involved with the patient and was visiting on a regular basis, despite her busy work schedule. She said that he behaved in a very immature way with her and seemed more like a helpless boy than a 30-year-old man.

In many ways, I thought that the pattern of breaking into women's houses and demanding sex had been re-enacted with the psychiatrist. Mr T appeared to have evacuated the usual worries and feeling about life into the external world and filled up his mind with a delusional system of his own creation. He lived inside this delusional world and projected any feelings of anxiety or depression about his situation out into the external world. His schizoid, spaced-out state was magnified by his use of marijuana. Mr T was then left feeling emotionally empty and detached from himself, lost in his delusion that he was Christ. He then presented himself to women in an attempt to excite their interest, in the hope that they would offer him a home. The underlying wish was that they would take him in and worship him by looking after him in an ideal way.

In her wish to help, the psychiatrist was also taken in, and taken over, by Mr T's search for a saviour who could take away all of his worries. In her countertransference, the psychiatrist became the saviour who could adopt the patient and provide him with everything. In the supervision group, we were able to think about the way the psychiatrist's commitment and compassion had led her to believe that she could adopt Mr T and save him from prison. Meanwhile, the patient had remained in a regressed state, projecting all responsibility for his care onto the psychiatrist.

Upon further discussion, it emerged that the psychiatrist's colleagues had discussed the case in some detail and did not think that the unit would be able to manage Mr T, because he had a history of absconding from mental health units and the magistrate had asked for some reassurance that the mental health unit would act as a place of safety. The mental health team did not feel that they could reassure the court that they would be able to contain Mr T. The psychiatrist was helped by the supervision group to separate herself from her powerful rescuing phantasy and to re-establish her clinical judgement and capacity to step back and think about the situation, including the limits of what could be done. She decided to stop trying to persuade her colleagues to admit Mr T. Instead, she thought about the possibility of contacting the psychiatric in-reach services and asking them if they could assess him, with a view to him being transferred to a forensic unit.

Discussion

These examples illustrate some of the reasons why mental health professionals need opportunities for supervision and reflective practice to talk about their work with patients in psychotic states of mind. They need the time to separate from the effects of the patients' communications and recover their capacity to think as themselves.

In our first example, the supervision group provided a space for thinking about the meaning of the patient's communication. In this forum, the supervision group leader encouraged staff to freely associate with the image of the man sitting on Ms R's head, and this enabled the staff team to put the missing emotion back into the patient's communication.

Jackson (1985) outlined the way in which concrete thinking leads to behaviour aimed at dealing with emotional problems by physical acts. The real nature of this type of thinking is often concealed by rationalization and presented as a perfectly reasonable course of action. In the second example, we can see how Mr S tried to persuade his CPN that he was a perfectly reasonable man with a perfectly reasonable belief that everything would be all right if only he could move away from these patients who were trying to drive him mad. At that point, Mr S was under the control of the psychotic part of himself—the part that believed that he could deal with his emotional problems through physical action. However, the real nature of the communication was concealed by Mr S's calm and reasonable demeanour. The CPN was partly pulled into a way of thinking that denied the patient's illness and began to think that the problems were not contained within the patient's mind but were, rather, contained within his physical environment. Although the CPN did hold on to some capacity to question what was going on when he said, "I do not understand what is going on", he became detached from his feelings and his capacity to use his clinical mind to question what was happening. For instance, he did not ask himself "why is this man in a hostel for people suffering from severe and enduring mental illness?" or "why does he think he is the only sane member of a mental health hostel?" or "why doesn't he think he would break down without medication and the support of the hostel workers?" or even "what is going on in relation to the other residents?" The CPN had been affected by the power of Mr S's denial and rationalization and cut off from his feelings, questions, and doubts about Mr S's request. In other words, he became detached from his capacity to think freely and take notice of his countertransference or "gut" reactions.

However, the CPN recognized that he "did not know what to make of" the presentation of Mr S and used the supervision group to help him recover his capacity for freedom of thought and to express his doubts and questions about the patient's thinking and mental state. The supervision group encouraged the CPN to reconnect with his feelings and start to examine the clinical picture in more depth. Towards the end of the first supervision session, the CPN said that he felt that Mr S was rather "intense and rigid" in his thinking. In other words, he noticed the feeling that everything would be all right provided that he went along with Mr S's way of thinking. As a result of a discussion, the supervision group was able to help the CPN to recover his identity as a mental health professional and reconnect with his feelings and professional judgement. This, in turn, helped him to make a more accurate assessment of the patient's mental state and the risk factors involved in the patient's care.

Psychotic patients often have difficulty in coming to terms with their illness and employ denial and rationalization to cover the extent of their psychosis. I have also found that some patients are particularly good at appearing to be sane and well despite the serious nature of their psychopathology. These patients also seem to be particularly effective at disarming mental health professionals' critical thinking and present themselves as reasonable and rational. When professionals join these patients in denying the seriousness of their psychopathology, it can lead to harmful or dangerous oversights in treatment and care. Mental health professionals need to remember that risk factors change according to the patient's mental state, and this can vary according to which care setting the patient is in. For example, in the case of a patient who is being cared for on an inpatient ward while being treated on anti-psychotic medication, the risk factors change radically once he has been discharged into the community and is no longer under 24-hour care or has stopped taking his medication.

In the third case study, the psychiatrist was affected by Mr T's wish to find a woman who would adopt him and offer him a psychic home. The psychiatrist's compassion and interest in the patient fitted with the patient's search for a woman who would care for him. She then became trapped in her countertransference reaction. The psychiatrist used the supervision group to help her to separate herself from the effects of the countertransference and to recover her clinical judgement. She was then able to establish a more realistic approach to the management of the patient.

Patients who suffer from a psychotic illness often communicate their distress, preoccupations, and concerns in complicated ways. Indeed, they may use actions or symptoms as well as verbal and non-verbal forms of communication. Communication takes place on an unconscious as well as a conscious level, and there are differences between psychotic and non-psychotic types of communication. Relationships are also used in ways that are difficult to understand, and patients may be wedded to destructive as well as healthy aspects of their personality. The difficult nature of psychotic communication can overwhelm mental health professionals, who feel tormented by the fragmented nature of the communication. This can be difficult to bear, and inevitably mental health professionals may try to keep the patient and his disturbance at a psychological distance. Indeed, without the necessary supervisory support, mental health professionals may become cut off and distant.

It is certainly true to say that anti-psychotic medication, which can take the edge off persecutory anxieties, forms an important element of treatment for psychotic conditions. However, shortage of staff and staff resources can lead mental health services into becoming over-reliant on medication. Indeed, anti-psychotic medication can sometimes be used by mental health professionals to keep the patient's disturbance at a distance. I believe that there is also a tendency to "over-value" the therapeutic effect of medication at the expense of other forms of therapeutic intervention: for example, the role of good nursing care and occupational therapy in a patient's recovery from a psychotic state is often minimized, with the therapeutic benefit of anti-psychotic medication over-emphasized. That said, I would reiterate that medication can be helpful when administered in conjunction with other therapeutic interventions.

The challenge of working with patients in psychotic states of mind is to get onto their wavelength and turn a psychotic monologue into a dialogue with meaning. For this to happen, staff have to remain interested in, and curious about, their patient's mind, and they have to risk being driven "mad" by a diabolical discussion with a patient, which may, in turn, leave them feeling mentally troubled.

Psychotic patients often communicate via concrete thinking or deadly delusional monologues (Segal, 1957)—forms of communication that have had the emotional life, and consequently the emotional content of the symbol, squeezed out of them. According to Richard Lucas (personal communication, 2009) mental health professionals need clinical supervision and space for clinical discussion to think about their psychotic patients' communications and their attacks upon their awareness of internal and external reality, and the effect of this on the professionals. A psychoanalytic assessment can also assist in kick-starting the process of tuning in to the psychotic wavelength of such patients and breathing life and emotional meaning into their deadly communications, as the next chapter argues.

CHAPTER SIX

The role of psychoanalytic assessment in the management and care of a psychotic patient

In this chapter, I argue that a psychoanalytic assessment can offer a dynamic picture of the deeper psychic structures in the patient's internal world, which underlie the presenting signs and symptoms of mental illness. This is particularly important with psychotic patients, who may successfully use denial and rationalization to cover up their underlying psychopathology (see chapter 5). The developmental perspective inherent in the psychoanalytic view can help clinicians to focus on repetitive patterns of behaviour. This is often helpful in deepening the risk assessment, as the best predictor of future behaviour is previous behaviour. The unstructured nature of the clinical approach and the emphasis on free association is designed to allow different elements of the patient's mind to emerge during the course of a psychoanalytic session. This information can then be used to provide a dynamic picture of relationships between different elements of the patient's mind and personality, including an understanding of what drives treatment-resistant aspects of the patient's mind, and to help construct a treatment and care plan designed to maximize healthy aspects of the patient's personality and minimize the risk of relapse.

Case example

The following extended clinical example of the psychotherapeutic assessment of a young man who had been referred to a specialist psychotherapy unit shows the way underlying unconscious processes manifest themselves in the relationship between the therapist and the wider mental health team. This patient masked the extent of his psychotic illness by presenting himself as someone who had suffered from a drug-induced psychosis in a way that undermined the treatment setting and the relationship between the specialist psychotherapy unit and the patient's local psychiatric team. The example shows the role of a psychoanalytic assessment for patients with serious psychotic conditions.

Mr U, a 26-year-old man with a diagnosis of paranoid schizophrenia, was referred to the psychotherapy unit by his community psychiatrist, as a result of a request from the patient. He had a history of mania and a delusional belief that he was Christ. Mr U had a sister two years older. His parents had separated when he was 5 years old, and their divorce had had a profound effect on Mr U; it was reported that he became angry and withdrawn. His father remarried and had three children with his second wife, leaving Mr U feeling rejected. Mr U was angry with his father for not showing enough interest in his upbringing. He was also angry with his mother—with whom he lived—for remarrying when he was 14 years of age, and during his late teens he became argumentative at home, until eventually his mother asked him to leave the house on account of his threatening behaviour.

Mr U had successfully completed several GCSE (General Certificate of Secondary Education) qualifications, but then he started smoking "skunk" (a strong form of marijuana) with a group of friends from school and dropped out of sixth form. Upon his first admission (under MHA section), Mr U said that he was putting different numbers together and gathering evidence that he was Christ. He also developed an obsessional belief that an ex-girlfriend—with whom he had had a relationship as a teenager—had betrayed him by having a relationship with a mutual friend. He believed that he would not have had his difficulties if she had stayed with him. Mr U had a history of stalking his ex-girlfriend, which eventually led to a court order preventing him from contacting her.

Mr U was seen within the context of a specialist psychotherapy unit for the treatment of patients with severe and enduring mental illness or personality disorders. Before agreeing to offer Mr U an assessment, the psychotherapy unit contacted the community psychiatric team and agreed to a joint care programme in which the psychiatric team would continue to monitor Mr U for the course of the extended assessment. In addition to a psychotherapist, each patient is allocated a keyworker from within the unit who has responsibility for liaising with the patient's local services.

The assessment

First meeting

Mr U was a handsome man but had a rather furtive air. At the first consultation he came into the room and immediately asked whether the pictures on the wall had been chosen deliberately "to test patients' reactions". Mr U went on to announce, in a calm, authoritative manner, that he had stopped taking his medication and did not feel that he needed to see the psychiatric team any longer. He presented this information in a reasonable way, as if it were of no more significance than telling me that he had decided to change his barber.

I said to him that I thought he was using the referral for psychotherapy as an opportunity to distance himself from the extent of his difficulties. He responded to my comments by smiling and saying that he had taken a lot of drugs when he was young, and he believed these drugs had damaged his mind. I said that I thought he preferred to blame the drugs rather than think about the problems in his own mind. I found myself getting increasingly worried that Mr U was relapsing and said to him that someone from the unit would contact his psychiatric team and ask for him to be seen as a matter of urgency. After the session, our keyworker contacted Mr U's CPN and communicated that we were worried that Mr U was breaking down. The CPN said he would phone Mr U and arrange a visit.

In the case of Mr U, we need to think of the psychotic and non-psychotic parts of his personality. Lucas (2009b) illustrated the way that the psychotic part of the mind attacks the sane part of the mind, projecting it into the external world or into the body. The psychotic part of the mind then tries to cover over the violence of the attack using denial and rationalization. The psychotic part of the patient's mind continues a secret existence, influencing the sane part of the mind, even though its influence may be disguised.

At the beginning of the session, the psychotic part of Mr U's mind projected his awareness of his difficulties, including his deceptiveness, into the therapeutic situation. He then covered over the actions of the psychotic part of his mind by acting like a man who was in absolute control of his life and mind. Mr U talked to me in the session as though he were quite reasonable in thinking that he was entitled to stop taking his medication and that he was ready to be discharged from psychiatric follow-up.

Second meeting

In the second assessment meeting, Mr U started talking about the regrets he had for the way he had been thinking and added that he knew he had to "keep a lid on" certain feelings. He went on to say his "paranoia" had done a lot of damage, and he had wasted many opportunities.

He also described how he sometimes felt that he was at the centre of everything and believed everything revolved around him. He likened this to the film *The Truman Show*, where he was the only genuine person. This struck me as interesting because, of course, the main character in *The Truman Show* falsely believes that he has control of his life when in reality he is totally controlled by others. I suggested that although he thought of himself as being at the "centre", he was not sure whether anyone else, including me, was genuinely interested. Mr U responded to this by saying that he sometimes thought he had "become the drug".

Moments later, he said that he did not like being seen on his way to his session because he felt that people would mock him for coming to therapy. I thought it was he who did not like seeing himself coming to his therapy, as he believed he was a special individual who did not need help. I reminded him of his grievance towards his father, who did not show enough interest in his development and left him to shoulder a lot of responsibilities. Mr U said, "Well, you can always blame your parents", to which I replied that perhaps he also blamed himself for being so weak as to need help. Mr U responded to this comment by doubling over in pain and saying that he felt lost. He then said that during the week he felt he was "being watched by eyes outside my flat". He went on to say that he felt lost in his own world and had gone to his mother's house and banged violently on the door until she had called the police.

Mr U appeared to alternate between psychotic and non-psychotic forms of thinking. When he said that he knew he had been paranoid and that his paranoid thinking had caused a great deal of damage, he appeared to be making a sane observation concerning the effects of the psychotic part of his personality. He showed real insight when he said he had to "keep a lid on" his feelings, because he could get carried away with his "brilliant" ideas and get lost in a psychotic world of his own creation. However, there was a further question as to how Mr U was using this insight: was it to help him think seriously about the nature of his difficulties? Or, was it to create an appearance of sanity in order to keep me away from more disturbing ideas?

Mr U had a deep-seated grievance towards both his parents for failing to put him at the centre of their preoccupations. It seemed that Mr U had been incubating a sense of betrayal and distrust since his father left his mother to start another family. Indeed, like Christ, he felt abandoned by his father, with the weight of the world on his shoulders. He also felt betrayed by his mother when she remarried during his teens, because he lost possession of her as an ideal figure. These adverse external factors, which were difficult and painful, disguised his resentment towards his parents for having a sexual relationship. Mr U would have liked to have inserted himself between his parents in order to control them. His envy of the parental couple found a home and expression in his grievance towards his father, for deserting him, and his mother, for failing to provide ideal care. I believe that his possessive preoccupation with his mother was then displaced onto his ex-girlfriend. I came to understand that his claim that he was "the only genuine person" involved a process of projective identification. Mr U projected his dishonesty and guilt into all those around him while adopting the posture of a "true man" or a peace-loving, genuine man. I think the reference to *The Truman Show* is also evidence of insight, as the psychotic system that controlled his life detracted from any curiosity or questioning.

Towards the end of the session, Mr U talked about feeling trapped inside his flat, with the eyes outside looking at him in an aggressive way; I think he was describing a momentary breakdown in his delusional system. It was as though he saw himself through these aggressive and persecutory eyes, as a broken-down man, abandoned and excluded from his mother's world. The eyes that looked at him in such an aggressive manner appeared to be elements of his sane self, aggressively projected through his eyes into the outside world, which then looked back at him in an accusing and persecutory way. In this instance, insight was felt to be an unbearable persecution, and he tried to break back into his mother's house as a place of safety.

Third meeting

A couple of days before the next session, Mr U's CPN contacted the keyworker attached to our service to say that he had phoned and arranged a time to meet Mr U, but when he got to the flat, Mr U was out.

In the third session, Mr U started by asking me whether the CPN had contacted me. He went on to minimize the significance of the missed appointment with the CPN, saying that it was a routine follow-up appointment. I said that I thought Mr U was trying to persuade both himself and me that he did not need psychiatric care and medication. He smiled and said that he had suffered from a drug-induced psychosis but had been studying numbers and felt that things were beginning to make sense. I said that I thought any understanding I might have developed had to compete with his genius for making connections.

On several occasions during this session, Mr U smiled discreetly to himself out of the corner of his mouth. I thought the smile indicated something slippery and deceptive, and I found myself becoming increasingly forthright in my comments—as if I were trying to pin him down or to force him to face reality. I told him I knew that he sometimes believed he was Christ. Mr U immediately said that he knew he was not Christ but then smiled and said, "but I am not the first person to believe they were Christ". He went on to say, "I just believe that things would be better if I could just talk to some people". I was sure this signalled that he was ruminating about his ex-girlfriend and might be in danger of breaking his restriction order.

After the session, our keyworker telephoned the consultant psychiatrist to inform him of our concern that Mr U was breaking down and liable to break his restriction order if he did not receive any psychiatric intervention and support. A week or so later, the psychiatrist phoned to say that he had assessed Mr U but could find no evidence of psychosis. He went along with Mr U's wish to stay off medication and said that he was beginning to question the diagnosis and wondered whether Mr U had indeed been suffering from a drug-induced psychosis rather than paranoid schizophrenia.

Mr U's capacity to conceal his psychosis and persuade the psychiatrist and psychiatric team that he was suffering from a drug-induced psychosis weakened the resolve of the psychiatric team to go on providing support for the psychotherapeutic assessment.

Fourth meeting

Mr U came to the fourth session in a very different mood, fluctuating between feelings of pain, humiliation, and mania. He said he had been to court, and the judge had warned him that he could be sent to prison as a result of breaking his restriction order. I was left confused about whether he had already broken his restriction order or why he had been called back to court. I said I thought that his preoccupation with his ex-girlfriend was imprisoning his mind to such an extent that he was likely to break his restriction order and end up in prison. He nodded sombrely and said that he had been to see the psychiatrist and requested some medication. I thought he was showing signs of some insight and taking the appropriate action.

Suddenly Mr U's mood changed; he started to describe a situation in which he was with a friend, who began smashing up a snooker hall. He talked about this in a calm and detached manner, incongruous with the level of violence described. I feared that neither the medication nor my interpretation were able to arrest his very disturbed mental state in any meaningful way. His mood then abruptly changed for a third time: he became quite excited, talking about the significance of certain numbers and hieroglyphs that revealed hidden meanings. As he was talking about this familiar subject, an equally familiar, vacuous smile came over his face.

At the beginning of the session, Mr U had appeared to be aware of the fact that his obsessive and delusional preoccupation with his ex-girlfriend could lead to his being sent to prison. When he said that he had been to see his psychiatrist and asked for medication, I thought that he was beginning to take some responsibility for his illness. I could feel his pain as the sane part of his mind realized he was in danger of losing control to his delusional preoccupation with his ex-girlfriend. This capacity to stay in touch with the insight and the disturbing thoughts and feelings about his broken-down state were unbearable, however, and so the pain of acknowledging his anxiety about himself was quickly followed by the violent story of a friend smashing up the snooker hall. I was shocked by the severity of the shift in his mental state and the terrifying power of the violent image of his friend. Leslie Sohn (personal communication, 2010) described the way psychotic patients are drawn towards dictatorial internal objects found within the psychotic part of the mind. These internal objects

provide omniscient and omnipotent solutions to emotional problems and thus protect the patient against the chaos and confusion
associated with psychotic breakdown. I felt that the patient with
whom I had been talking at the beginning of the session was gone.

Bion (1957) described the psychotic patient as struggling in a
never-ending conflict between the life and death instincts. In the
situation outlined above, Mr U smashes up his awareness of reality,
which can bring him so much pain. Mr U's mental state is fluctuating between moments of insight and psychotic denial. The violence
of the attack of the psychotic part of the mind on the non-psychotic
part destroys his ego's capacity to think. In this fragmented state
the ego has no capacity to repair its functioning and consequently
resorts to the magical repair provided by a delusional system. Mr U
retreated into his world of numbers and hieroglyphs. He protected
himself from awareness of the destruction of his mind by searching
for evidence that he was Christ—a peaceful figure who provided
the world with meaning. Again, a member of the unit contacted
the psychiatric team, alerting them of our concerns.

> Several days later, Mr U failed to turn up to his appointment. A
> member of our service contacted Mr U's consultant psychiatrist,
> who informed us that Mr U had been remanded in custody after
> breaking his restriction order. Several days later, a probation
> officer telephoned me to say that she had interviewed Mr U
> following his arrest. She said that he had become increasingly
> bizarre as the interview progressed, and she was worried that
> she had made things worse by asking Mr U questions.

Mr U seems to have been able to hold himself together and disguise
his disturbance during the course of a relatively short and structured mental state examination based on the presence or absence
of symptoms. The probation officer's interview and more in-depth
approach to the offence penetrated beneath Mr U's defences and
revealed his underlying psychosis. As the psychosis was revealed,
the probation officer was left feeling that she had damaged Mr U
and undermined his apparently coherent state of mind.

> Several months after starting his custodial sentence, Mr U's
> in-reach psychiatrist from the prison contacted our service to

say that he was being transferred back to his local psychiatric service. Apparently, Mr U had become floridly psychotic while in prison, and the prison authorities decided that he needed to be transferred back to the mental health team. Mr U responded quickly to the inpatient-ward environment and anti-psychotic medication. Within a few weeks, the team talked about a discharge plan and asked the head of our service if someone could attend a professionals' meeting to discuss his case. Mr U had improved considerably during his stay on the ward and had responded well to anti-psychotic medication. The plan was to discharge him on a standard-level CPA to the local recovery centre, where short-term care is provided for patients in the community.

In the subsequent meeting, I pointed out that although Mr U's mental state had improved, he was dependent upon the setting to provide him with care and treatment. I drew attention to the way in which Mr U's identification with Christ, "the epitome of forgiveness and peace", concealed an aggressive and possessive attitude towards his ex-girlfriend. Indeed, this aggressive preoccupation with his ex-girlfriend was likely to re-emerge as soon as he stopped contact with the psychiatric team and the psychosis re-established its grip upon his mind. Mr U needed to be cared for within the context of a treatment team who understood the long-term nature of his illness and were prepared to hold responsibility for his care. This would include an on-going risk assessment and management/treatment plan.

I was subsequently contacted by a senior clinician within the CMHT who said that a new care plan that took my assessment of Mr U's needs into consideration had been developed. He had been moved from oral to depot medication and had been referred to an Assertive Outreach Team (AOT) on an enhanced-level CPA, a more intensive level of care. As a result of breaking his restriction order and the risk he presented, he had also been referred to Multi-Agency Public Protection Arrangement (MAPPA), who monitored his treatment in conjunction with his psychiatric team. Several years later, I followed up Mr U' s case and found that he was still being cared for by the AOT and MAPPA, and he continued to receive psychiatric follow-up and treatment on an enhanced-level CPA. There had been no further admissions or reoffences, and he had started to become involved with some sheltered work.

Segal (1950) outlined the need for a particular clinical setting that supports the psychotherapeutic treatment. She emphasized the need for access to inpatient facilities, which allow the treatment to continue in the event of the patient being admitted to hospital. She also made the point that a failure to establish a sufficiently robust setting often contributes to the failure of the treatment.

Discussion

Patients in psychotic states of mind are continually drawn away from the emotional demands of external reality and into the world of their psychosis. The negative symptoms represent a pull towards a deadly psychotic organization and away from contact with internal or external reality, and patients need mental health professionals and relatives who are able to help them to resist this through engaging them in activities and interactions that provide an anchor in external reality. Richard Lucas described this social network as the "exoskeleton" surrounding the patient (Lucas, 2009a), which comes under attack at times from the psychotic part of the patient. Mental health professionals have to be able to withstand these attacks and hold on to their long-term clinical view. The patient needs a team of clinicians who are working together in the interests of their treatment and care. The clinicians need to communicate on a regular basis about the patient and be able to endure a certain amount of anxiety. An active attempt to involve the patient is required, even if at times this goes against the patient's wishes. Problems can arise when the patient's denial or rationalization influence the clinician's thinking and undermine the clinical container. Lucas (2009d) has shown how the power of the communication can affect the clinician, evoking powerful countertransference responses, which can push them to ignore the degree of disturbance and inappropriately settle for a more ordinary or neurotic explanation for a patient's behaviour. A study by McCabe and colleagues showed that consultant psychiatrists avoided patients' direct comments and questions about their psychotic symptoms in psychiatric consultations (McCabe, Heath, Burns, & Priebe, 2002).

By requesting a referral for psychotherapy, the non-psychotic part of Mr U was searching for someone who could think about him and his difficulties. However, at the same time, the psychotic part was using the referral to disguise his psychosis by presenting himself as a neurotic man who could not get over the breakup with his ex-girlfriend and had experienced a brief drug-induced psychosis. The patient's controlled presentation helped to disguise the real extent of his illness, and he succeeded, at least temporarily, in causing a split between the psychiatric team and the psychotherapist. Mr U's promotion of the view that he was suffering from a drug-induced psychosis, rather than a schizophrenic illness, further weakened the clinical container necessary for treatment. It may also be true to say that his comment that he "was the drug" represented his recognition of the powerful hypnotic effect he had upon clinicians. In many ways, Mr U was continually repeating the offence by breaking into the minds of others and interfering with their freedom to think. He did this by posing as a peaceful man concerned to find out the truth. The reality was that while the sane part of his mind might have wanted the psychosis to be uncovered and arrested, the psychotic part of his mind was determined to keep everyone in the dark by concealing the truth.

It is also worth reflecting on the patient's comment that he sometimes thought he was in an episode of *The Truman Show*. This was an important communication. In the film, Truman is unaware of the fact that he is living on a film set and the producer is controlling his world. Mr U was living in a delusional world of his own creation, and his mind was controlled by his psychosis. The identification with Christ suggested an attempt to cover and deny the violence of his internal world and his wish to control the parental couple. He presented himself as the person who had come to save his mother and ex-girlfriend from the corrupting influence of other men. Meanwhile, the grudge and the controlling nature of the relationship with his mother and ex-girlfriend were concealed.

This case illustration shows how an extended psychoanalytic assessment of patients with a serious psychotic illness can assist in their psychiatric management and care. Minne (2003), working in a forensic context, has also shown how psychoanalytic understanding makes a crucial contribution to the assessment of risk. The psychoanalytic assessment of Mr U provided a valuable insight into his psychological makeup and its relationship to his offending behaviour. The assessment gave a dynamic and more realistic picture of the risks involved in the care of Mr U. These risks were difficult to detect in the more structured setting because of the powerful countertransference feelings he evoked, probably at an unconscious level, in those working with him. Indeed, Mr U was able to promote an idea that he had suffered from a transient psychotic disorder, rather than the more difficult reality of longstanding schizophrenic illness. Denial and rationalization were used to cover over the effects of the psychotic part of his mind. The reality was that as soon as he was discharged from psychiatric care and stopped taking his medication, his mind became more vulnerable to psychotic thinking. He would then start to listen to the delusional system in his mind; he became obsessed with his ex-girlfriend and in danger of breaking his restriction order. However, in a straightforward mental state examination, he was sane enough to know that he had to keep a lid on his psychosis so he could keep his psychotic thinking quiet while answering leading questions during assessment.

As is often the case, my fuller understanding of Mr U consolidated with the benefit of hindsight. However, I believe that there needed to be this level of thought about him because any relapse was likely to lead to him breaking his restriction order, with potentially severe consequences for both him and his victim. The psychotherapeutic assessment helped to establish an appropriate psychiatric management plan or supporting treatment structure that met his needs more adequately. This reduced the risk of relapse and reoffending behaviour and also seemed to lead to an improvement in Mr U's functioning. The "exoskeleton" Mr U required to support the non-psychotic part of his ego was represented by the enhanced level of CPA, depot medication, and referral to multi-agency public protection arrangements. The management of his illness was no longer left solely with Mr U; rather, it was shared with mental health professionals who carried responsibility for his treatment and compliance with medication.

As Lucas says, a psychoanalytic framework can help mental health professionals and management alike to understand the psychotic process and tune in to the psychotic wavelength (Lucas, 2009e). Although psychoanalytic treatment may not be appropriate for some patients who suffer from a psychotic illness, it does provide a model for thinking about unconscious as well as conscious communication. It also provides a model for thinking about the way relationships and repeated patterns of behaviour are used to communicate underlying feelings, conflicts, and anxieties. In this case, such thinking could be provided through offering a psychoanalytic assessment alongside the treatment provided by the psychiatric team.

CHAPTER SEVEN

Deliberate self-harm: "I don't have a problem dying, it's living I can't stand"

There are patients who communicate their psychological difficulties through persistent and serious self-harm; this may, at times, involve visible attacks on the body or dangerous, life-threatening behaviours. Many of the patients who act in this harmful way will deny the serious nature of their self-harming and may mock others' concern. As long as they are alive while they play the game of "Russian roulette", the life-threatening nature of their actions can be minimized. Anxiety about the threat to life or the damaging nature of the behaviour is often projected, leaving the responsibility for keeping the patient alive with family, carers, and/or the mental health services. This can cause torment for those who carry responsibility for and have a duty of care towards a patient who can treat his life in a careless or reckless way, and he can also be rejected by mental health services because he is either thought to be too risky or deemed to be untreatable.

Many, though not all, patients who harm themselves have had neglectful, disruptive, or damaging relationships with their primary carers, and their internal worlds are often inhabited by hostile figures that attack and undermine their sense of well-being. Understanding patients' relationships with their bodies is central to understanding their relationship with themselves and their internal objects. Patients who harm themselves often project onto their skin as a way of registering their feelings about themselves and others. Indeed, their skin often provides the evidence of their damaged relationships with their primary objects. Bell (2001) describes the way these patients locate the bad object in the body, which is then attacked. The body may also represent hated aspects of the self, and the anatomical part of the body attacked often has significance and meaning.

Freud said that the ego was primarily a body ego: "The ego is first and foremost a bodily ego: it is not merely a surface entity but is also the projection of a surface" (1923b, p. 26).

Klein believed that the infant has introjected the loving and caring relationship with the primary object, forming a fundamental building block of the infant's ego and good sense of self, which then has the capacity to bear anxiety and psychological pain, enabling the infant to develop a mind capable of thinking about itself in relation to the external world. This sort of ego can bear to think about painful emotional states as it does not fear annihilation and fragmentation. However, the infant that has an inadequate, neglectful, or bad relationship with the primary object may develop an ego that can only evacuate unwanted or painful feelings. This over-reliance on projection interferes with the capacity of the infant to assess itself in relation to others.

Bion (1962a) showed that failure of containment in early life led to the development and internalization of an ego-destructive superego—a murderous structure that hates the psychological pain associated with meaningful relationships or emotional links and employs primitive defences designed to deny and evade psychic reality, rather than to learn and adapt. Instead of a mind that supports the individual in thinking about the relationships between the self and others, the individual develops one devoted to evacuating painful aspects of the internal world, either into the external world or into his body.

Case example

My treatment of a patient, Ms V, was on the outer limit of—and possibly beyond—what is manageable in an outpatient psychotherapy setting. During the course of the treatment, she and I struggled with a murderous, psychotic object that dominated her mind. This defensive internal structure, based, I believe, on a fundamental failure in Ms V's relationship with her primary object, used self-harm to enhance omnipotent defences by projecting feelings and thoughts into the body, where they could be disowned and attacked; it alternated with a sadomasochistic defence against trauma and loss. I outline some of the difficulties I had managing my own strong countertransferential reactions in the face of pressures generated by the clinical situation; anxiety about the extent of Ms V's risk behaviour undermined at times my ability to maintain the analytic setting.

When the treatment began, Ms V was in her mid-twenties, with a 14-year history of self-harm by cutting, severe overdoses, and anorexia. Despite these difficulties, she did quite well at school before undertaking an artistic training. Ms V's early twenties were marked by promiscuous sexual relationships and heavy drug use. She had received various psychological therapies and outpatient psychiatry over the years. In the meantime, her self-harming behaviour had increased, and she started to take overdoses on a regular basis. Ms V was assessed for psychotherapy and was diagnosed as having severe personality disorder, underpinned by a psychotic internal object. The assessor referred Ms V to the psychotherapy service, where she was offered twice-weekly psychoanalytic psychotherapy.

Family history

Ms V was an only child born to a married couple, who were part of a fundamentalist religious sect. When Ms V was 2 years old, the family adopted from the sect an older girl, called Jane. According to Ms V, Jane's behaviour was anxious, and she was a demanding child, who became more behaviourally disturbed during her teens. Ms V felt that Jane's behaviour began to dominate the household, and her father became increasingly involved in trying to look after her. Ms V described her mother as a cold woman who left the family when Ms V was 12 years old and who had not been seen since. Ms V felt that Jane had "wrapped her father around her little finger", as he was always doing things to alleviate her anxieties and destructive behaviour. She said that she thought her father had thrived on Jane's psychological disabilities and her consequent dependence on him. Ms V also said that she was made to feel guilty as a child and remembered a priest from the sect telling her that Ms V's success at school made Jane feel worse about herself. The priest also told Ms V that she was the devil's child, and on one occasion he conducted an exorcism. Her memory was that her father had supported these actions.

At the commencement of the therapy, Ms V was single, although she occasionally had casual sex with men. Ms V maintained her artistic work, although this was impeded by her self-harming behaviour.

Therapeutic setting

Because of her high risk of suicide, Ms V's case was managed jointly between the specialist psychotherapy unit and her local psychiatric services. Patients treated in the unit were offered twice-weekly therapy for two years, followed by an open-ended group. Her case was discussed at unit meetings on a regular basis, particularly when there was an escalation in her self-harming or risky behaviour. The clinical nurse specialist and the responsible medical consultant attached to the unit kept in regular contact with the local psychiatric service for the duration of Ms V's treatment.

During the two-year course of her twice-weekly psychotherapy, Ms V had to be admitted at times under a mental health section, either as a result of an overdose or because of the seriousness of her self-harming. The therapy was put on hold during the admission and then restarted post-discharge. Ms V resented these admissions; she said they interfered with the two positive things in her life: her work and her therapy.

Early stages of the treatment: making contact

When I first started seeing Ms V, she described a sadistic voice in her mind that demanded she should harm herself. When I tried to take up the way she distanced herself from any responsibility for the severity of her self-harming behaviour, she would mock me, saying that her body was meaningless. At this stage in the therapy it was sometimes difficult to locate any part of Ms V that would register or admit to anxiety or concern about the damage being done to her body. Indeed, the part of the patient that was worried about the abusive relationship with this tyrannical internal object was projected into me.

On one occasion early in the treatment, Ms V came into the session telling me that she had cut into her abdomen the words "fat cow": "as that is what I am". I said that I thought Ms V hated all appetite or desire, as it made her feel vulnerable and weak. She mocked this comment, saying "why would I want to desire anything that would make me weak?" I suggested that part of her must be terrified of this murderous internal voice that demanded she do so much damage to herself. She said that her skin was as thick as a crocodile's and could not be damaged. I said that I thought the skin covering her underlying sensitivity was this cold murderous attitude she had towards herself and her body—a part of her that despised ordinary needs and desires. Ms V contemptuously replied that she found the thought of needs or desires disgusting. I said that she wanted me to take responsibility for her self-hatred and self-harm. I also thought that another part of her was worried that one day the self-hatred would either wittingly or unwittingly kill her. Ms V was quiet for a minute and then started to talk about a character in a book having a pang of regret while committing suicide. I said she withdrew from the pain and desire for life, into the clutches of the murderous internal figure that mocked her attempts to reach out to me. She started to cry and said that too much damage had been done, and she was no longer human.

In the initial stages of the therapy, Ms V tried to maintain her view that there was nothing wrong with her way of thinking, as she lived inside, and was identified with, this highly destructive mental state. Ms V's mind was dominated by a murderous, psychotic internal voice that forbade any ordinary desire or need for an object relationship. The voice demanded devotion to the omnipotent power of self-harm and self-hatred. Ordinary non-psychotic feelings of attachment or involvement represented a threat to the psychotic part of her mind, and consequently these were attacked. The desires, appetites, and needs were projected into her body, where they could be controlled, disowned, and sadistically attacked. Even so, no matter how much damage she did to her body, the voice inside her head mocked her for never doing enough: "Do you call that a cut? That's not a cut, that's a scratch; I don't know what all the fuss is about." The non-psychotic part of her mind that was aware of the damage she was doing to herself and the terrifying nature of her self-harming behaviour was projected into me. As the therapist, I felt pushed into one of two positions: either I accepted my relative helplessness and adopted a passive stance in which I stood back and witnessed the horrifying effects of her murderous self-hatred, or I became very active in interpreting the sadistic attacks on her body and life, in an attempt to inject some concern into her.

Rosenfeld (1971) described the way destructive narcissistic structures in the mind function like a pathological gang, offering a retreat from the pain of reality through the use of an omnipotent psychic mechanism to deny reality, rather than face it. This destructive internal structure seduces the individual into believing that loyalty to the structure will be rewarded by protection from the pain of loss, dependency, conflict, and vulnerability. Rosenfeld outlined the way parts of the internal gang promise to deal with the individual's problems in a pain-free way by employing manic defences of triumph, control, and contempt.

Ms V dismissed all the aspects of her mind associated with

desire and attachment, as well as other unwanted elements that needed to be projected and controlled. She felt that any desire, love, guilt, or jealousy made her vulnerable to the world of attachment, and she could then be hurt.

Attack on the body as an expression of her hatred of her mother

I believe Ms V's absent relationship with her mother was reflected in her hateful relationship with herself and her femininity. She hated anything that made her think of herself as a baby or as a mother. She attacked her breasts and vagina because she wanted to remove any idea that she was a woman with a female body. She hated her breasts—"because the thought of a baby sucking on a breast is disgusting"—and her vagina because it represented somewhere where penises could get into her and give her a baby, "which was monstrous".

Ms V told me that she had sex with men who were abusive towards her and who were unable to form a relationship with her, usually because they were involved with somebody else. I thought these sadomasochistic relationships represented repeated attempts to master and control her experience of childhood trauma. She was traumatized both by her mother's distance and lack of interest and by Jane's displacement of her as her father's favourite. In phantasy, she momentarily triumphed over Jane and her mother by stealing a figure representing her father from another woman.

These sadomasochistic relationships were also represented in the way she saw herself as a sexual object: from time to time she would attract men who, she believed, found her damaged and scarred body attractive. She thought that all of her scars represented vaginas that could be penetrated. In this way, Ms V attacked and undermined the specificity and creativity of her genitals. In phantasy, she created a picture of herself as a sort of sexual pincushion that could be used only for abusive sex, but not for the sort of intercourse that could lead to the creation of a baby or to a loving relationship. Ms V believed that any man attracted to her had to be perverse in his interest in her damaged mind and body—"What normal man would be attracted to me? I look like Frankenstein's Monster." Thus she was permitted libidinal feeling and desires, provided that they were imbued with hatred and sadism. In the transference, I took up her belief that I was the man with a perverse interest in her damaged mind and body.

The use of the skin as a means of communication

The amount of scarring visible to me in sessions varied during the course of the therapy. At times, Ms V would cover up; at others, she would wear clothes that revealed scarring on various parts of her body. I took this as part of the clinical presentation designed to communicate various things at different times. In some sessions, I believe I was meant to be shocked or horrified. In others, I was given a visible and concrete reminder of her damaged self, which would evoke more sympathy and concern for the extent of the damage. During the early stages of the therapy, Ms V also used the sight of her thickened scarring to enhance the view of herself as an impenetrable figure with crocodile skin. At times, it was difficult to locate any sane part of her that could be anxious about the effects of her terrifying self-hatred.

Bick (1968) outlined the way infants use their skin to hold themselves together and provide a boundary when they feel they are falling apart. She described patients who had difficulty establishing a secure internal ego and consequently developed what she called a "second skin"—often orientated around a skill or talent—to enhance their feeling of integration and identity. When patients scar themselves in a significant way, the skin becomes a visible and concrete representation of a damaged sense of self and evidence of a damaged and damaging relationship with the primary object. It is as if the individual is saying, "Look, rather than having a good sense of myself and a good internal ego, I have internalized an object that hates me." Indeed, the scars of this battle between one part of the self and another are written all over the skin, providing a visible record of the internal relationship. The thickened skin also seemed to represent the withdrawal of the patient into an identification with an ego that did not feel that it could afford to let very much in or out that was not controlled by the patient.

We can see Ms V's identification with the child who felt completely unloved and unwanted. She wanted to attack the body she had been given as a way of providing visible evidence of her parents' lack of care and neglect. Who would have a child who would do such a thing to the body she had been given?

After the initial few months of therapy, there were moments when Ms V was able to separate herself from the psychotic internal structure. Her underlying sensitivity and vulnerability became much more evident. This change was also evident in her view of herself and her relationship with the therapy. Towards the end of the first year, Ms V described me as "a whaler throwing harpoons into a whale, then following it until it eventually becomes exhausted and drowns". This change in image provided an accurate picture of the changing clinical situation. Ms V felt that the therapy was weakening her allegiance to the destructive internal gang, and this made her more vulnerable to painful emotions in the therapy. I thought the whale represented the murderous superego being weakened by my interpretations. However, this posed its own threat, as neither of us knew whether she would survive without her omnipotent defences. My image of myself was as an ancient whaler in a small boat that could be sunk by one swish of the whale's tail.

This image of a vulnerable boat that could be sunk at any moment chimed with my feeling about developments in the therapy. Ms V's relationship with the therapy had, I believe, started to support and strengthen the non-psychotic part of her mind. However, the development of this part of her mind also drew attention both to the extent of damage to her mind and body and to guilt about the damage done, and despair about the possibility of repair sometimes forced her back into the hands of sadomasochistic or psychotic defences. Ms V's relationship with the therapy also threatened her relationship with her murderous internal object, and she described the way painful emotional contact in sessions would lead to a demand that she harm herself. It was as if the internal structure demanded to see evidence of her loyalty to the gang. Indeed, the more emotional contact there was between us, the more we both feared reprisals on the part of the murderous internal object.

Re-enactment of historical traumas in the transference

Powerful communications can have an effect on the therapist's countertransference and may induce the therapist to re-enact aspects of the patient's past.

Occasionally during the therapy, Ms V had to be admitted to hospital as a result of extreme, life-threatening self-harming behaviour. After her first period of admission, Ms V returned to the therapy in a cold mood, complaining that the admission had been a complete waste of time and had interfered with the therapy and with her work. She was witheringly contemptuous of the hospital staff and their attempts to help her, while also accusing them of being incompetent and uncaring: "I could have done anything to myself in there, and no one would have stopped me."

I was criticized for "letting her go" and was made to feel that I had been more interested in protecting my own professional reputation than the therapy (as I did not want to answer for a suicide). In addition to feeling that I was the target of her scorn, I was accused of being weak and unable to manage her murderousness and my own anxiety. I was grateful to the psychiatric team for giving me some respite from the constant anxiety that Ms V would kill herself, and I felt provoked by her withering disdain. I said that I thought the extent of her murderous attitude towards herself forced others to take responsibility for her, but that, while I had a role to play, ultimately she was the only person who would be able to keep herself alive and protect the good things in her life. In effect, I was reminding her that she had brought the admission upon herself with her destructive behaviour. Ms V said she felt I was saying that she was not taking her therapy seriously, and that I would prefer to see another patient. She reminded me that she had recently thrown away large quantities of tablets that she had been hoarding for an overdose, and she complained that she did not feel that I understood how hard she was struggling to control her self-destructive impulses.

In listening to this, and on reflection, I became aware of the way I was unwittingly re-enacting a traumatic aspect of Ms V's childhood by accusing her of being the demon child. In the face of the therapy's impotence against the terrifying and awesome power of the murderous and psychotic internal structure, I had turned to my own version of an omnipotent religious solution as I exhorted her to exorcise her demon. It was as if, in desperation, I had been taken over by a wishful phantasy that Ms V could split off and discard the destructive aspect of herself, allowing the healthier part that was capable of forming a relationship with the therapist to flourish. Although I hoped that over time she might take back responsibility for the management of her destructiveness, I did not believe that in her current state she was capable of that for anything more than short periods of time. In hindsight, I could see I was trying to force Ms V into becoming more reasonable and responsible, because I found it hard to bear the reality that Ms V could destroy any good developments in herself or good intentions in me.

Breakdown in the treatment setting

About halfway through the therapy, I reminded Ms V that the therapy would end in a year's time, and I gave an actual date for the ending. Although this announcement led to an increase in her acting-out behaviour, it did not completely destroy the contact and work we were able to do together.

During one of our sessions soon after my announcement, Ms V said I was like an ambulance crew walking away from the scene of an accident. This statement hit me hard, as I really felt that I was walking away from a car crash and leaving her life on a knife-edge. Ms V said she was upset about missed opportunities and found herself thinking about the amount of damage she had done to herself over the years. She was not sure that she could bear the pain of acknowledging what had been lost. Ms V said that she wished she had come to see me many years earlier. Then there was a change in mood, as Ms V seemed to become more anxious. When I said she thought I was walking away from her in a smashed-up state, as if I did not believe anything could be done, Ms V started to cry and said that she could not be expected to manage her own murderousness and self-hatred. I said that I understood that this frightened her, as she worried that without my help she would not be able to resist the frightening power of her destructive internal voices. Ms V said that she sometimes thought she might as well be dead; she feared she would end up like Mrs Rochester, stuck in an attic endlessly harming herself and attacking anyone who came near her. I said that I thought the struggle and anxieties of living could always be trumped by the attraction of a pain-free existence. It was as if the deadly voice in her head promised to deal with all the pain of life through death. Ms V said she had a persistent daydream about drifting off into a narcotic dead sea.

Several weeks after this session, Ms V announced that her relationship with her psychiatric team had broken down, and she had been discharged. In the session, it became evident that Ms V had become increasingly scathing and contemptuous of the psychiatric team's attempts to help. I think the sadistic part of her mind wanted to leave me entirely on my own with the anxiety about her risk and responsibility for her behaviour. This seemed like a repetition of Ms V's early childhood, with the parents splitting, leaving the father to deal with Ms V and her adoptive sister. Following a discussion in the unit clinical meeting, it was agreed that the consultant and the clinical nurse specialist would try to engage a new psychiatric team who could help us monitor her risk and who would admit her to hospital if absolutely necessary. This all took some time, which left us trying to manage the psychiatric risk on our own. During this period, Ms V would sometimes hint at some act of self-harm, which she would not disclose. This left me feeling uncomfortable, as she had already told me of her long-term suicide plan. It was quite clear to me that she was a serious suicide risk, either by mistake or design. Without consciously changing my role into a more psychiatric approach—something I would normally do if I thought this was appropriate—I sometimes found myself unwittingly moving away from my analytic stance of free-floating attention and into a more active approach, as I focused on her relationship with the psychotic and destructive aspect of herself. However, I think my changed approach in response to my own anxieties about her self-harming behaviour actually contributed to an escalation in Ms V's cutting and overdoses. Eventually a new psychiatric team was able to assess and admit her for treatment and care.

On her return to therapy, after several weeks' break, Ms V said that she felt that, before her admission, I had become completely preoccupied with her self-destructive behaviour and had given no support to the healthier part that was trying to live. She said: "I don't have a problem when I'm harming myself, I find that comes naturally. However, I do have a problem knowing what to do with myself when I'm not self-harming or thinking of suicide." She added that she thought I had to leave it up to her whether she lived or died. She said my focus on her self-harming left no room for any helpful treatment.

We can see Ms V's childhood history being re-enacted in the therapy, as the non-psychotic part of her that wanted help and support in her struggle with the murderous, psychotic internal object felt let down when I did not recognize her efforts. Although I could not ignore the self-destructiveness, I believed Ms V was saying something helpful when she drew attention to the fact that the noisy, self-destructive part of her dominated the treatment sessions at the expense of a part of her that wanted to progress and develop. However, responsibility for the self-destructive state was often projected into and located in me while Ms V provoked me to take action. The internal and external support was also attacked and ridiculed, as she wanted to pull me into trying to rescue her from her murderous self-destructive behaviour. The relationship between us was being watched and monitored by the murderous internal object. If this object felt I had been provoked into trying to rescue Ms V, it would demand that she then increase the intensity and level of acting out.

In her paper "Envy and Gratitude" (1957), Klein said: "In dealing with this anxiety [that prevents integration] one should not underrate the loving impulses when they can be detected in the material. For it is these which in the end enable the patient to mitigate his hate and envy" (p. 226). Again, on reflection, I could see the way my preoccupation and anxiety about the power of her relationship with her self-harming behaviour represented a re-enactment of her father's erotized relationship with her adoptive sister Jane. Her secretiveness and coyness were used to pull me into an erotized, anxious, preoccupied relationship with the destructive aspects of herself, which left her healthier parts unrecognized and unsupported. The wish to split the psychotherapy treatment from psychiatric support was related to the patient's wish to cut my relationship with her internal and external good objects. In the transference, I was being "wrapped around my patient's little finger" by the part of her that was identified with Jane, while the part that struggled to get on with living was ignored and left to fend for itself.

> The consultant and clinical nurse specialist from the unit met with the new local psychiatric service, and a care plan was put into place to continue the therapy until its conclusion and then transfer Ms V's care to the local personality disorder service, because she said she would not attend any treatment group offered at our unit. This plan was discussed with Ms V, and she was encouraged to continue meeting with the psychiatric team in the meantime.

As a result of Ms V's helpful feedback and the unit discussion, I was able to re-establish an analytic stance and state of mind based on free-floating attention. I started to tune in to the subtle ways the non-psychotic part of the patient would make contact with me. During this phase of the therapy, the delicate relationship between the psychotic and non-psychotic parts of her mind became more apparent. I began to understand that Ms V could be allowed to develop positively, provided that the psychotic part of the gang was not too provoked. I thought Ms V could make use of the therapeutic setting as long as I could resist the temptation to either, on the one hand, rescue her from her self-destructive internal state or, on the other, to become cut off and blasé about the seriousness of her risk. In order to help me to keep the therapeutic frame, I needed good external support from psychotherapeutic psychiatric colleagues.

Negative therapeutic reaction

When Ms V sensed that I was trying to tune in to the subtler communications emanating from the non-psychotic part of her mind while ignoring the more destructive elements of her personality, she became extremely anxious that this would provoke an attack from the internal gang. In one session, Ms V told me she had received very good feedback for a piece of work and then suddenly found herself in A&E after taking a serious overdose. We can see this life-and-death struggle between the part of her that was trying to make use of her capacities and opportunities and the influence of the destructive narcissistic gang. I was reminded of the priest who made her feel that her development was at the cost of her adoptive sister, Jane.

In her paper on the negative therapeutic reaction, Riviere (1936) describes the way patients undermine developments by destructive acting out. I realized I had to acknowledge that the destructive part of Ms V was always present and prone to feeling enviously excluded, especially if there was some healthier contact made in the therapy. Destructive self-harming behaviour could always triumph over ordinary anxieties and pain.

Ms V's progress in the therapy would often be followed by serious life-threatening acting out and subsequent admission to hospital. On returning from her third admission during the course of the therapy, Ms V continued her usual complaint about the admission being a waste of time. I responded by saying that although these breaks in treatment were upsetting and disruptive, there was very little we could do about it apart from trying to re-establish the working relationship as quickly as possible. I also said that at certain times, when Ms V's mind was taken over by the murderous and destructive aspect of her personality, her life was at risk and we had to take this threat seriously.

The problem of mourning and the end of the therapy

In the last year of therapy, we discussed the possibility of Ms V moving on to group psychotherapy, as is the usual practice with the unit, but she did not feel she could manage a group. I believe that her difficulty in contemplating moving to a group was related to her feeling that she had been deprived of a good internal object that could support her. Ms V did not believe she could bear sharing the therapist with other members of the group.

In the last few months of treatment, Ms V said she feared that having an ending imposed upon her would drive her to act out in a brutal way. She decided to finish at a time of her choosing, thus taking control over the ending rather than having another traumatic loss inflicted upon her. As planned, we then transferred all of Ms V's care to the local service.

Discussion

Ms V's extreme self-harming and repetitive suicidal behaviour provided an intoxicating, omnipotent internal solution to avoid the pain of traumatic situations and life. Indeed, the propaganda that accompanied the self-harm was designed to make me believe that Ms V was unreachable. It was as if she were saying, "Any individual who has so little concern for herself or her life and can inflict so much damage cannot be hurt or reached." The daily game of "Russian roulette" also allowed her to believe that she controlled life and death by either bringing death nearer or pushing it away. In this way, she secretly told herself that she would triumph over loss and the facts of life.

At times, when the psychotic internal gang was in the ascendancy, the sane self was projected into the body, where its influence could be controlled, disowned, and attacked (Lucas, 2009b). In this state of mind Ms V communicated her internal conflict by action. She feared that I would listen to her propaganda and conclude that the therapy was useless, and she would be left with no sane ally, the victim of an endlessly murderous, internal structure—the madwoman in the attic who has nothing to do but endlessly harm herself in a repetitive way, killing life or anything of value.

The sane and healthy part of the patient was often projected and disowned, but if it had a voice, it might say, "Please don't believe the propaganda of the psychotic part, please don't give up on me and leave me on my own with that murderer." The evidence of this internal conflict was represented and recorded on Ms V's skin, which provided a historical record of the battles fought and the damaging cost of the internal war.

There was always a particular issue that needed to be addressed after an admission. This related to my capacity to re-establish and

maintain a psychotherapeutic setting in the face of Ms V's provocative and risky self-harming behaviour, which could provoke
me into shifting from the listening and interpretative function of
a psychoanalytic approach to the more active approach involved
in a psychiatric examination and risk assessment. At times when
this happened, I thought it was related to a genuine fear that the
murderous aspect of the patient would eventually triumph and
she would kill herself. At other times, I think it was used to nudge
me into an active psychiatric stance and to temporarily give up
my analytic position of focusing on the meaning of Ms V's communication. This was designed to undermine my attempts to think
about her at a symbolic level, and her provocative comments could
be used to pull me into a sadomasochistic relationship. If I failed
to respond to provocative comments about self-harm, she could
accuse me of being blasé, unmoved, and detached from the seriousness of her risk; however, if I became more active and psychiatric
by asking questions, she believed that I had been overwhelmed
by anxiety and resorted to action designed to reduce my anxiety.
Although she desperately needed my help, it provoked envious
attacks from a part of her that was committed to her destructive
internal structure.

After one admission, Ms V told me she had always had to look
after everybody, including Jane, her father, and even her mother
before she left, as she had felt they were not capable of looking after
themselves. If Ms V witnessed examples of my acting out because
she felt I was too quick to turn the session into a psychiatric consultation or to break the frame, I think she worried that I could not
face the extent of her omnipotent destructiveness and had turned
to a version of therapeutic omnipotence out of desperation. Ms V
said that her self-harming behaviour drove people mad, and she
thought she had control over other people, as she could make them
do bad things. She described herself as living with a wrecking ball
that attacked any life or development. She now feared that any
discussion of her destructive feelings would lead to me calling the
psychiatric team and asking for them to admit her.

During Ms V's treatment, I often felt impotent in the face of the
terrifying strength of her self-harming and suicidal behaviour. I
was affected by the power of her murderous internal structure and
harboured a continuous fear that she would kill herself. Leslie Sohn

(personal communication, 2010) described the way in which psychotic parts of the personality form identifications with dictatorial figures that offer violent solutions to painful emotional problems. This powerful communication, which was sometimes enhanced by the sight of Ms V's scarred body, had a profound effect on me in the countertransference. Anxiety caused by the very real threat to Ms V's life, as well as the threat to positive developments made through her involvement with the therapy, led to me abandoning from time to time the analytic attitude of "free-floating attention", as I was taken over by a desire to cure or rescue the patient from her terrifying situation. Ms V's portrayal of herself as the victim of her self-destructiveness nudged me to act as if I believed we could deal with the problem of her destructiveness by splitting it off and projecting it. In this state of mind, any improvement was based on an artificial division between the healthy and destructive aspects of the self, followed by projection in phantasy of the unwanted aspects of Ms V's mind. This omnipotent solution provided both the patient and me with temporary relief before the projective solution inevitably broke down and the self-destructiveness returned. Although this manic reparation provided some respite, it denied painful questions about the reality of Ms V's internal world and her reliance on destructive aspects of the self. At times, I was nudged into acting as a mentor who could help get rid of these destructive internal structures. The painful fact was that she was not just the victim of this destructive aspect of the self: her murderousness was protecting her from psychic pain by attacking any creative relationship developing between us.

The painful reality for both Ms V and myself during the course of the therapy was that we had to live with both sides of her personality—the part that wanted to live and develop, and the part that wanted to punish and destroy. All I could do in therapy was to describe the nature of her internal relationships and the way they undermined her capacity to make emotional contact and develop. Ms V's internal oedipal structure consisted of an absent mother who, she believed, would have preferred that Ms V did not exist—I believe this formed the basis of her murderous internal object—and a father whom she engaged in a sadomasochistic relationship. In this structure, there was very little support for Ms V as a person in her own right. This configuration was re-enacted in the transference, as I was felt to be either a cold, indifferent maternal object or an over-involved phallic father who was trying to rescue her from her abusive internal structure while wrapped around its finger.

Although Ms V often encouraged me to act out by pushing or provoking me in one direction or another, she was also helpful in pointing out when I had lost the frame or acted out, and her comments helped me to re-establish an analytic stance. These comments emanated from the sane part of her mind that desperately needed a therapist who was able to maintain the therapeutic setting. This included a balanced state of mind that was not overwhelmed by anxiety and was able to reflect on material without jumping to conclusions. I needed to be able to listen to the material with free-floating attention, while holding the different parts of the patient in mind. I also needed to be able to step back from the interaction and observe my own reactions and part in the process. An additional problem related to the patient's perverse use of the relationship to torment and punish me. Most of the time it was difficult to know what part of the patient was communicating at any given moment, and I would become aware of the way I might have acted out only on reflection and through discussion with colleagues after the sessions.

Caper (1997) outlined the need for therapists to have a secure relationship with their internal objects that will help them to resist the pull towards either rescuing patients or resorting to a paranoid-schizoid, narcissistic fusion with them. A realistic, depressive patient–analyst contact as a proper object helps patients to establish proper contact with themselves.

I relied on the support of the unit in thinking about the clinical situation, in order to help me to maintain—and at times to recover—the analytic setting; this also depended upon the link with local psychiatric services that helped to assess and manage the very real risks. The establishment of a setting that could manage the patient's disturbance when she started to act out in a serious and life-threatening way was an essential part of the treatment. Ms V's attempts to split the relationship between the psychotherapy and psychiatry services related to her wish to attack and undermine my relationship with a structure that helped me to maintain my analytic stance. When she was successful in her attempts to cause a breakdown in the setting, she would become both excited and hateful but also anxious that her omnipotent defences had succeeded.

Ms V fought hard to be referred for psychotherapy, and she maintained that, for her, it was a lifeline. However, the severity of her acting out and the inconclusive nature of the ending leave unanswered questions about the efficacy of this treatment. Although the therapy was anxiety-provoking, disturbing, and on the edge of what was manageable in an outpatient setting, Ms V nevertheless maintained a view that it was productive. In her paper "Relating to the Super-Ego", O'Shaughnessy (1999) describes the treatment of two patients whose minds and ego functioning were dominated by a relationship with a pathological ego-destructive superego. She emphasizes the important role therapy played in helping the patients to separate from the pathological superego through contact with the normal superego in the encounter with the therapist. I was left in no doubt that Ms V made meaningful contact in the therapy and achieved a degree of separation between the psychotic and non-psychotic aspects of her mind. This allowed her to develop and strengthen a non-psychotic part of her mind that was able to register realistic concern and worry about herself; this, in turn, exposed her to guilt and anxieties about the damage done, which, she feared, would provoke a savage backlash from the murderous internal voice. I also think she developed an awareness of the way she used sadomasochistic relationships as a defence against the pain of depression and guilt about damage she had done to herself, as well as damage that had been done to her earlier in life by others. However, these developments were fragile, and Ms V believed she needed on-going individual treatment in order to support her.

The ending of the therapy left us both uncertain whether Ms V's life instinct and fragile internal good object could resist the terrifying power of her destructiveness.

CHAPTER EIGHT

Anorexia:
the silent assassin within

norexia nervosa is a serious psychiatric illness, characterized by an inability to maintain an adequate, healthy
body weight. The prognosis for most cases of mild anorexia is good, as patients recover and go on to lead ordinary lives.
However, anorexia nervosa remains the psychiatric diagnosis with
the highest mortality rates, and a significant proportion of those
diagnosed either go on to become chronically ill or die as a result
of the physical complications of starvation and low body weight.
Steinhausen (2002) showed that only 46% of patients fully recov-
ered from anorexia nervosa, a third improved with only partial or
residual features of the disorder, and 20% remained chronically
ill for the long term. A low body-mass index, a greater severity
of social and psychological problems, self-induced vomiting, and
purgative abuse have all been identified as predictors of poor out-
comes in this disorder. The chronic patient group can be difficult
to treat because they can be extremely persuasive (plausible), and
the full extent of their disturbed thinking and actions is not always
evident. Indeed, the fanatical control of their objects and aggressive
attacks on life is often denied. This mental state can have a powerful hypnotic effect on mental health staff and/or relatives, as the
patient may try to persuade them that her actions and thinking are

understandable, natural, and normal. In reality, the patient's mind may be in the grip of a murderous psychotic process determined to starve her of life in order to control it, rather than live it. The extent of the manic triumph and contempt for life—and the help such patients need—is often hidden beneath an exterior of calm rationality. The reality is that, in more severely ill patients, the anorexic object controls the patient's mind and can function like a silent but deadly assassin.

Freud (1911b) thought that in very early life the infant is dominated by the pleasure principle, which dictates that the infant seeks pleasure and avoids pain. He described the developmental task of the infant in terms of a shift from the pleasure principle to the reality principle. As the frustrations of reality gradually impinge, the infant is forced to acknowledge and come to terms with the restrictions that external reality places upon it. The job of the maturing ego is to seek a compromise between the need for instinctual gratification as represented by the id and the prohibitions of external reality as represented by the superego.

Klein (1946) believed that this process begins when the infant discovers that the breast it depends upon for goodness and life is a separate object, outside its omnipotent control. She thought the capacity of the infant to bear this developmental step is linked to the internalization of a "good" object through the contact with the breast, which then forms the core of the infant's internal world. This object gives the infant a good feeling and helps it bear the pain and anxiety associated with separation and dependence. When the infant has difficulty internalizing a good object, it may try to deny separation by employing primitive defences, which involve distortions of reality. Klein described how the infant uses projective identification to sustain a phantasy that it controls or possesses the breast, thus avoiding a separation. Projective identification involves a phantasy in which part of the ego is projected by the subject into the object. When it is used in a flexible way, it forms part of normal communication, providing the imaginative leap by which we are able to put ourselves into someone else's shoes. We usually describe this as empathy. However, when it is used in an inflexible way, it can become pathological, as, in phantasy, aspects of the self are disowned and forcibly projected into others.

Bion (1962a) developed Klein's ideas through his theory of the relationship between the "container" and the "contained". He described the way the infant used the mother as a "container" for indigestible psychic material, which he described as the "contained". In this process, the infant communicates its distress to the mother through noises or actions. In phantasy, the infant has projected its psychic material into the mother. If the mother's response is in tune with the infant's projected state of mind, the infant re-introjects its projection after the mother has done psychic work on the communication. Over time, the infant internalizes the mother's capacity to contain and think about undigested psychic material. This is the basis of a "good" relationship between mother and infant, and it paves the way towards separation and development. "It may develop, if the relationship with the breast is good, into a capacity for toleration by the self of its own psychic qualities" (Bion, 1962b, p. 118). If, however, the infant's communications/ projections are either not accepted by the mother or the infant's relationship to the mother is disturbed by too much envy, then this benign circle breaks down. The infant experiences this as an attack by the mother on its link with her and feels its communication has been stripped of meaning. The infant develops a mind that is threatened by psychic pain and forced to evacuate any awareness of emotional meaning. Emotional links are hated because they represent a connection between the infant and an external object, confronting the infant with the reality of separation and its dependence upon others, which an infant with a fragile ego is unable to manage.

The result of such an experience in infancy is shown in the case of a patient, Mrs W, who suffered from a serious and chronic anorexic illness, and whom I treated in twice-weekly individual psychotherapy. The full extent of her addiction to this destructive internal structure did not become apparent until her first breakdown. It also became clear that I was affected by the powerful nature of the patient's non-verbal communications as, from time to time, she pulled me into a *folie à deux*. This way of relating provided her with reassurance that the threat of the therapy had been neutralized by her control. However, the cost was that it denied the patient the real but disturbing emotional contact she needed

in order to develop and progress. At times, these countertransferential feelings interfered with my ability to make the painful
emotional contact needed in order for her to develop.

Case example

Clinical history

Mrs W was a 26-year-old patient referred for treatment to a psychotherapy unit by a consultant psychiatrist attached to an eating
disorders unit. Patients in the unit were often offered twice-weekly
psychoanalytic psychotherapy for two years, followed by group
psychotherapy. Mrs W's treatment was managed jointly between
the unit and the eating disorders team. Mrs W came from a wealthy
middle-class family. She described her father as a rather pathetic,
obsessional man, who drank too much and never stayed in one
place for any length of time, and her mother as obsessed with her
own looks; she said her mother had once accused Mrs W of stealing a younger boyfriend.

Her parents had divorced acrimoniously when Mrs W was 8
years old; she stayed with her mother and two younger brothers
until she went to boarding school at the age of 10. Mrs W had
always felt her mother to be self-obsessed, and she described being
neglected during her early teens while her mother went on a manic
spree. She reported long-standing difficulties with food: when she
was 8 years old, she remembers a voice in her head telling her not
to eat because she was greedy. At boarding school, Mrs W developed a phantasy that she was pregnant as a result of kissing a boy,
and consequently she ate minimal amounts of food to stop herself
from gaining weight. She developed anorexia in her early teens and
had several admissions to hospital in her early twenties. Despite
her difficulties, she achieved several A Levels before going on to
complete a degree at university.

Mrs W married in her mid-twenties. However, at the time of
coming for therapy, the marriage was in difficulty, as her husband
wanted a sexual relationship and children. Mrs W told me that
although she had had sexual relationships in the past, these were

one-night stands or casual relationships. She did not enjoy sex with her husband and was terrified of becoming pregnant, saying, "The thought of having a baby inside me is disgusting." Indeed, the whole idea of becoming a mother was frightening, as a result of her own disastrous maternal relationship.

The therapy

Mrs W said she hated coming for therapy because it made her feel greedy and bad for having problems. She found the therapy extremely difficult, but she attended diligently and placed great importance upon it. The sessions were characterized by painful communication issues, as Mrs W talked very quietly, and her speech was fragmented. She rarely had any expression in her voice and would start sessions by saying three or four abstract words that appeared to be detached from any sort of reality, then fall silent while waiting for my response. If I did not respond, she put great pressure on me to speak, complaining that I was punishing her or making life difficult. She once said that she did not mind what I said, as long as I said something. Mrs W complained that I was making her talk, which was an adult activity and not to be trusted: "People say one thing and do something different." She preferred to communicate through art or action, which she saw as more trustworthy. She described an internal voice that warned her not to tell me too much, as I was "dangerous and not to be trusted". In his paper "Attacks on Linking", Bion (1959) described the way the links with the good object, which the infant depends upon for life, are split up and enviously attacked. I think Mrs W was unsure whether I was a good object that she could relate to or a seductive and unreliable object that she should keep at a distance.

At times, I felt tortured by the demanding nature of the communication difficulty, as Mrs W would watch and scrutinize my every move. She perceived silences, breaks, or changes in the setting as a threat to her link with me, and she would often look around at me from the couch to see what I was doing. She once explained that if I did not speak, she then assumed I had turned into a harsh, critical figure; consequently she had to look at me to confirm I had not. Mrs W insisted therapy was meant to be different from her life experiences, and when I was silent, I was repeating the traumas of the past, in which she was made to feel invisible by her parents. Mrs W believed that therapist and patient should be perfectly in tune, in a way that denied any difference between them. She saw me as an ideal and god-like figure of her own creation who expected her to submit herself to the therapy in a devoted and submissive way. For example, she often tried to imagine my opinion about something and then felt under pressure to fit in with my view. When she could not do this, she would keep her actions to herself, fearing my disapproval.

As a result of the demanding nature of the communication, I sometimes found myself either leaning towards her because she mumbled, or amplifying what she had already said. On a few occasions, the tormenting slow nature of her speech made me finish her sentences. I sometimes felt as if I wanted to pull the words out of her. In this situation, I was the one with the desire and need to know what was going on in her mind, hungry and at times greedy for information. Mrs W believed the aim of therapy should be to make her feel secure and loved in a way that her family had not. She put pressure on me to act in an omnipotent way by insisting that I should know what she was thinking and feeling, without having to be told. When I did not comply with her pressure to make interpretations based on very little information, Mrs W complained that I was feeding her deep-seated insecurities.

Birksted-Breen (1989) highlighted anorexics' failure to separate psychologically from their mothers as one of the main clinical features of the illness. She described how anorexics oscillate between the fear of separation, which is equated with abandonment, and fears of being engulfed. Patients may try to minimize the issue of separation by talking quietly and secretively, therefore pulling the therapist towards them, as Mrs W did with me.

Mrs W hated separations and breaks in the therapy, as she felt that she no longer existed in my mind. John Steiner (personal communication, 2015) described the way certain patients acted as if mother's love was equivalent to a material with physical properties, a finite resource that would run out when used up. In the transference, Mrs W acted as if there were a competition for my interest and care between her and others areas of my life. Indeed, in breaks she often developed a strongly held belief that my wife was pregnant and assumed I would be too worn out to work with her when I returned and consequently would end the therapy. It was as if she thought I could look after only one baby, as two at the same time would be too demanding. Mrs W's physical state and perception was dramatically affected by the breaks, and she regularly complained that her eyesight had deteriorated. After one break, she told me her optician had recorded a marked change in her eyesight, which he could not explain. He had recorded her as being short-sighted during the break, but a second test when therapy resumed revealed her sight had returned to normal. Mrs W became anxious that I would no longer recognize her or forget I had ever seen her.

Clinical material

This first clinical example is of a session that took place just before the first break. During the previous session, Mrs W had complained she was too compliant, and she had wanted to stay on the couch at the end of the previous session to see how I would react.

Mrs W was silent in the early stages of the session. She then spoke in a quiet, lifeless voice. She felt that in the previous session I had got her where I wanted her and had then left her to cope with the rest of her day, and as a consequence her day was ruined: "When I cycled home, I had this feeling I wanted cars to crash into me. I wanted to be smashed to bits." [Pause.] "Then I had this problem with my eyesight. I could not see properly. I kept walking into people, but I'm worried about going to the optician, because they will say, 'You are making it up'. It's as if I'm a ghost, and no one sees me until I bump into them." I said that she thought I could not see the way the sessions had robbed her of her sight and her capacity to see. Mrs W replied by telling me that she had gone to a Tai Chi class with a friend: "I only went for a bit of fun, but I became frightened because I could not take in anything the instructor was doing with my eyes."

Mrs W said she felt I didn't care: "It doesn't make any difference to you does it? Nothing ever changes. You are unaffected by me. You are trained to be unaffected, so that if I kill myself, it is my responsibility. I think if I was hit by a car and admitted to hospital, you would see me if I could come to the sessions, but not if I couldn't. I sometimes have this fantasy of tearing my skin in front of you to see how you would react." I said that Mrs W wanted to make me understand the unbearable pain of feeling that I was wedded to my method in a way that made her feel I was not interested in the pain of her situation.

Mrs W tried to overcome the problem of my separate existence by establishing an illusion that I was an ideal therapist, with no characteristics other than those she ascribed to me. She often justified this by telling me that I was supposed to be a blank screen that she projected things onto, and consequently she "had to think of me as a woman". If she thought of me as a man, I became a threat, "as men are only interested in sex". She assumed I would want to be thought of as a female therapist, because women have breasts and can feed and support their infants. Mrs W put pressure on me to provide a womb-like experience, where there was no separation or need to communicate. Any separation from this state left Mrs W in a state of panic, as she felt she felt she no longer existed, she became the ghost I could not see, while at the same time she lost contact with the parts of her mind that had been projected into me. In relation to the material about the Tai Chi, I thought Mrs W was telling me that she had come to the therapy only as a bit of fun, but the therapy made her painfully aware of the fact that she couldn't take things in through her eyes. I also think Mrs W thought that I was the instructor who seemed to be unaware of the fact that my pupil could not follow my elaborate moves or take anything in. I was the impenetrable object that was wedded to my theories and immune to her pain and suffering. The picture of her standing in front of me and tearing her skin conveys her feeling that she has to tear herself to bits in front of me to get anything through and concretely show me what is inside.

Britton (1989) developed Bion's container–contained theory further by describing the impact of the oedipal situation on the mother–infant dyad. Britton maintained that this psychological step becomes bearable when the infant has been able to internalize a relationship to a "good" breast that helps it tolerate and think about its experience. However, if the infant has not successfully internalized a "good" breast, then the appearance of the oedipal situation feels like a premature intrusion. The infant's capacity to bear the pain of the oedipal situation can be arrested if the parental couple intrude before the infant has established a relationship with a good breast that can respond to the infant's projections. "Faced with the oedipal situation the psychotic mutilates his mind" (Britton, 1989, p. 37). It is no coincidence that Oedipus blinds himself with Jocasta's brooch. Steiner (1990) points out that Oedipus "attacks his eyes, which are the link to the reality he cannot bear, and he tries to annihilate the source of his pain by destroying his capacity to experience and perceive" (p. 229). The idea that Mrs W would crash into someone represented both a destruction of her mind, which was so painfully aware of her predicament, and an attempt to violently re-enter her object, as if existence outside the object was unbearable. What was so dramatic was that her eyesight, as well as her insight, was affected: the eyesight that offered the physical evidence of my separateness and difference was destroyed.

> Shortly after the first break, Mrs W's weight dropped, and the eating disorder team decided to re-admit her under section. She complained of an obstruction in her bowel, which caused considerable pain when she ate, and consequently she refused food. She accused staff of making her worse when they encouraged her to eat, and she demanded to be transferred to a medical ward. Once in the general hospital, and despite the presence of nurses from the eating disorders unit, she was given nil by mouth and fed through an intravenous drip. Mrs W repeatedly accused staff of abusing her by feeding her via the drip. Indeed, she interfered with her drip and tried to pull the needle out of her vein. The eating disorders ward manager responsible for Mrs W's psychiatric care said she did not like asking the nurses to do one-to-one observations because she felt as though the staff were being forced to witness the victory of death over life. No physical cause for Mrs W's pain was found, and she was transferred back to the eating disorders unit, where she eventually began to improve.

During this time, I thought Mrs W's mind was dominated by an anorexic internal object that hated any desire or dependency upon another person. This structure did not acknowledge the need for anyone or anything else outside the self but believed, instead, that the problems of life could be dealt with by denial of need and fanatical control. The anorexic internal structure attacked ordinary needs and desires, craving self-sufficiency, starvation, and death in preference to desire and life. After several months with the support of the eating disorder unit and a low dose of anti-psychotic medication, Mrs W was discharged from hospital.

The breakdown of the treatment on this occasion made me review my approach as, on reflection and with the help of clinical discussion, I realized that I had underestimated the influence of this anorexic internal object that prevented Mrs W from taking anything in. Indeed, just after her return to therapy, Mrs W told me about a dream that demonstrated the influence of this internal structure. In her dream, *Mrs W was in a therapy session with me, but behind her, in the corner of the room and out of sight, was a dark, gangster-like figure that controlled what she could or could not say to me.*

Sohn (1985a) describes the way anorexics make greedy demands upon the object to offer things but then enviously attack what is offered, as if it was no longer what was wanted. The object is made to feel as if it has offered something unappetizing: a cold meal. Interest then turns to the next interpretation—the next meal. By forcing therapists to believe that they must keep trying to find the ideal meal, as this will be the one that will provide nutrition and satisfaction, patients attack and undermine therapists' potency and creativity. In addition, patients also enviously spoil the part of them that is hungry and available for contact. Lucas (2009c) described the division between a psychotic anorexic internal structure that hates any need or desire for an object and the non-anorexic part of the mind. These two forces fight for supremacy within the individual's psyche.

Mrs W's dream gave an accurate picture of the internal figure that controlled the therapy and contact with me, a gang leader that forbade her dependence upon me as a separate object. This anorexic internal object represented Mrs W's control of any appetite or desire for contact between us. The breaks were such a threat because she also feared that her envious controlling attitude deprived me of any satisfaction, which would mean that I would lose interest and be desperate to get away from her. Lawrence

(2008) described anorexics as being addicted to omnipotent control over internal and external objects. They want to create an objectless world in which they are free from feelings of separation, jealousy, and envy. A destructive part of the self attacks and undermines any attachment to life or any part that remains hopeful. At the same time, the aggressive attack on life is denied by rationalization.

Caper (1997) points out the way patients' primitive communications elicit an immediate identification within therapists. Although this is an important step in any therapy, he argues that there is a danger that therapists slip into an identification with the patient that prevents them from thinking about the communication. "The analyst tends to fall spontaneously into a countertransference illness as part of his receptivity to the patient's projections, and he must cure himself of it if the analysis is to progress."

I could also see the way I had been tempted to compete with Mrs W's addiction to this deadly anorexic structure by offering omnipotent understanding. For instance, in the face of Mrs W's torturous and fragmented communication, I would sometimes find myself filling in the gaps, assuming that I understood something she was saying or making premature comments based on too little information. In this way, I unconsciously acted out in the countertransference as my omniscience tried to fill in the gap between what had been said and what I understood. The effect of this dynamic was to take over the desire for contact between Mrs W and myself. This sort of false contact acted as a *folie à deux* that provided the appearance of therapeutic contact while actually depriving the therapist of a patient and the non-anorexic part of Mrs W of the psychological nutrition she needed. The reliance on assumptions in the communication with Mrs W avoided both the reality of separation between us and the pain of emotional contact. If we communicated as two separate individuals with our own minds, we might find out painful things about each other that did not fit in with the fantasized ideal. Indeed, the ideal therapist she developed in her mind could only be maintained if I functioned in an omniscient way. This bypassed the need for the painful and humiliating process of verbal communication. As she once said to me, "Adults words are not to be trusted; it's actions that count."

During the intervening months, I tried to tune in to the influence of this internal structure by interpreting the way the anorexic part of Mrs W's mind attacked any desire or need, thereby depriving her of help. At other times, when she was more available, I took up the way she would present the material and then withdraw back into an anorexic state of mind, going cold on the contact. I tried to resist the temptation to get too interested or excited about material, which would have allowed her to retreat into an actively passive stance. Instead, I tried to keep an eye on her involvement and withdrawal and interpreted the way desire for communication and understanding was projected into me. This change in stance led to a change in the nature of Mrs W's communication, as she became more animated and lively in sessions. She also told me that she had started drawing and described her art as providing a commentary on the therapy. The separation between Mrs W and myself and the symbolic nature of the communication provided me with more of a picture of Mrs W's internal world.

The next session described took place a few months later, just after the Christmas break. I had recently changed the time of the session from outside normal clinic hours to a daytime appointment. Mrs W's phantasy was that I was spending more time with my wife—who, she thought, had just had a baby—rather than coming in to see her for her session.

Mrs W started by saying that she was angry with me about the previous session, which, she thought, had been a waste of time: "I felt like you were saying that you did not know me. . . . On Friday I just felt furious, because I wanted to be here with you, not at home with my husband. But I am not allowed to do that, am I? Just lie here next to you—but it is not allowed in here, is it? You just want to talk in the here and now." I replied by saying I thought Mrs W felt deprived of a special relationship with me where she could cuddle up to me and keep me to herself. Mrs W said she had been drawing and wanted to show me: "But it is a waste of time, isn't it, because you are not interested? You will not want to see the drawings; you will want me to talk." I said I thought Mrs W was wedded to non-verbal communication, which bypassed the need to put things into words. She wanted to be allowed to cuddle up next to me as a way of avoiding thinking together. Mrs W became extremely upset and replied: "Yes, well, what good are you? I feel like you are trying to diminish your position in my eyes. I feel like leaving and not coming back. What is the point in coming?" I said I thought Mrs W did not feel able to control the sessions when she was required to describe her feelings and thoughts.

She went on to describe the drawing, which was of a king and queen looking into each other's eyes, and below them was a small green figure with a stake through her heart. "It is so obvious, I do not need to explain. That is how I feel: stuck outside, separated, of no consequence, like a witch." I said I thought the anorexic part of her felt betrayed and wounded when we were communicating. Mrs W said that she just wished I would leave her alone and get out of her head: "You do not do anything for me." Mrs W said my approach made her feel as if she did not exist: "I feel so childish, so upset, but I fear that if I get upset, you will turn to stone." I thought that she was saying that she feared that if she criticized me, I would respond by going completely cold on her. Mrs W said the voice that told her not to talk to me was getting louder, but she realized she did not have to listen.

In this session, a shift in Mrs W's internal world was reflected in the way she communicated in the therapy. The drawing showed an internal battle between the anorexic and non-anorexic parts of her mind. At the start of the session, Mrs W described her continued wish to pull me into an idealized relationship, based on non-verbal communication in which we should cuddle up to one another rather than talk and think. This pressure was accompanied by an accusation that the therapy was cruel for expecting a damaged infantile figure, such as Mrs W, to communicate verbally in an adult way. She also justified her preference for non-verbal communication when she argued that verbal communication was not to be trusted, "as people say one thing and do another". Although Mrs W complained bitterly, she then went on to give a vivid verbal picture of her internal world and her relationship with the therapy and me through her description of the drawing.

This represented a shift in the patient's internal world and a shift in Mrs W's relationship with the therapy. If we think of the drawing as a dream, we can see the way it works on several levels. On one level, the description of the king, queen, and small green figure represent the struggle in the patient's internal world. Mrs W was describing the way shifts in the therapy were beginning to kill off and weaken the influence of the anorexic part of her mind. Mrs W continued to demonstrate the effect of this change by saying that although she could hear the anorexic voice in her mind, she didn't have to listen to its influence. This indicated that the non-anorexic part of her mind was beginning to separate from the anorexic part and find its own voice. On another level, the separation from the anorexic part reduced her omnipotent control of me as a therapist; this allowed the emergence of the oedipal picture, which Mrs W believed would be a disaster. Mrs W hated coming across any evidence of my being supported by relationships with analytic figures in my internal world. She believed that this would lead to a shameful exposure of her psychological difficulties.

In his paper "The Missing Link", Britton (1989) described patients who lack a good internal object as believing that holding on to and controlling any external good object is a matter of life and death, and that the emergence of the oedipal situation threatens their relationship with the ideal object and, thus, their relationship with the object that keeps them alive.

Segal's (1957) differentiation between a symbolic equation, thought to be the object, and a symbol, known to represent the object, is described in detail in chapter 1 (see "Symbolization and concrete thinking"). It is only with a shift towards symbolic thinking, in which the difference between internal and external reality is realized, that separation becomes bearable. The symbol is felt to represent the object internally and is not confused with the real external object.

Aggressive thoughts and feelings in phantasy do damage to the symbol rather than in reality. Symbols, felt to represent the lost object internally, are used to help the process of separation. Mrs W was faced with the loss of her relationship with an ideal object—a therapist who would cuddle up to her in an attempt to deny the need for separation and thought. The therapy became a sort of psychic womb that protected her from the pain of life and living. It was also designed to protect her from the pain of development. Mrs W believed that the loss of this relationship was a disaster and led to a form of psychic annihilation. The psychic separation also

introduced the idea in the patient's mind of the therapist's relationship with a third object and the oedipal situation, which, in turn,
provokes violent feelings of rivalry and hatred.

The king and queen who are staring lovingly into each other's
eyes perhaps represented Mrs W's feeling that the non-anorexic
part of herself was developing a relationship with the therapist.
The witch-like figure represented the anorexic part of her mind,
which denied and despised any appetite or desire for contact and
felt that the progress in the therapy threatened its omnipotent
control over the patient's mind. Mrs W's drawing also represented
her psychic conflict. Separation from the object and a reduction in
her reliance on omnipotent control allowed her to develop a more
mature, engaged, straightforward relationship with the therapy,
providing an opportunity for development but also allowing the
emergence of the oedipal situation, which, Mrs W believed, would
kill the omnipotent infantile self she had always relied upon to
control her objects and keep her alive. The thought that I would
turn to stone if she expressed her feelings was, I believe, related to
the fear that I would not be able to bear her criticisms, frustration,
and disappointment in me and my limited capacity to understand.

Over the next few weeks, Mrs W talked increasingly about her
art and told me that an art dealer friend of the family had asked if
he could display some of it. Mrs W angrily told me that this was
not possible, as the therapy was too influential in her work and the
infantile nature of her difficulties would become visible and public
in a humiliating way. I said that I thought I was the art dealer who
was inviting her to display her thoughts, feelings, and desires in
the therapy and that part of her wanted to do this. However, she
also felt ashamed of her desires and wishes and feared they would
not be received and understood.

This session took place several months later, just after I had told
Mrs W that the therapy would have to stop in one year's time.
Not surprisingly, Mrs W was extremely upset; she felt that the
end of therapy would be a catastrophe and would leave her
in a terrible and unbearable half-improved state. She was also
convinced that it was a condemnation of her as a hopeless case
and worried that it was related to the extent of her dependence
upon the therapy.

Mrs W started the session by telling me that she felt so anxious she didn't think she could cope: "Last night I lost my sight. It has not happened for a couple of years, but it is frightening. I think I should either get some medication or stop coming. My vision was in pieces, broken up like a kaleidoscope. It's all to do with you telling me that you are going to stop my therapy. I don't know if I can bear it any longer. My level of anxiety is too high. Also I have stopped doing my artwork." I thought she worried that neither of us could deal with her feeling about the loss of the therapy. Mrs W then told me that she had pains in her cervix and that she had arranged for a gynaecology consultation because she was convinced she needed a hysterectomy. I thought she felt I was leaving her with the anorexic part of her mind that hated life and wished to rip out any desire or creative potential. I thought she needed me to understand that this destructiveness was provoked by the announcement about the end of the therapy.

After a pause Mrs W said: "Everywhere you look, there are programmes criticizing psychotherapy." I said that perhaps she thought my failings should be broadcast. The therapy had identified various problems and interfered with her usual way of doing things, and I was leaving her when there was still more work to be done. Mrs W said: "Since I told you about the artwork, you have been trying to get away." I said I thought Mrs W thought I hated to hear about her needs and the intensity of her involvement with me. Mrs W said that when she lost her art, she lost her capacity to see, but I said that while she felt that describing her feelings was humiliating, she was also aware that she needed me to understand what was going on so that I could help her. Mrs W then said: "My aunty told me that when I was a baby I used to leave my mouth open when I was feeding: I used to refuse to suck when I was a baby or chew when I was a small child. The liquid or food would fall out of my mouth, and this would really upset anyone feeding me."

Not surprisingly, the announcement about the end of the therapy caused Mrs W enormous anxiety and pain, and there was a corresponding deterioration in her capacity to communicate verbally.

The threat of the hysterectomy was designed to really hit me, as Mrs W threatened to rip out the means of creating life. Williams (1997) described the "no-entry" system of defence, designed to keep the object out, developed by anorexic patients. It was as though Mrs W were saying, "Well, you have attacked any hope of further creativity. I'm back in the hands of the anorexia, and I'm blocking off one of the ways you have been able to get inside my mind."

The controlling anorexic object, which had been pushed into the background by therapeutic work, returned to the foreground. Mrs W's thinking was taken over by concrete, psychotic solutions to neurotic problems. In the transference, the sexual organs represented the non-anorexic part of the patient that desired contact with the therapist—the part that was emotionally available and seeking to make things grow inside her. However, when faced with the pain and loss associated with the end of therapy, the anorexic part of her mind offered a concrete solution—to remove the organs that contain the desire and return to a sexless, desire-free, infantile, narcissistic state of self-sufficiency. Any development that had come about as a result of Mrs W taking things into the non-anorexic part of her was treated as if it were a contaminant rather than a developing idea. The internal babies resulting from the therapy were attacked.

The propaganda of the anorexic part of the patient's mind is that by creating a perfect, objectless world in which one doesn't desire or need anyone or anything else, one can avoid all the pain associated with dependency and loss. Indeed, a phantasy can develop that one can control life and death, even though in effect all one can do is bring death nearer and then push it away for a time.

In this clinical example, in response to the shocking reminder of the end of therapy, Mrs W became concrete in her thinking. There was also a sense of her desperately trying to communicate something about her fear that the end of the therapy felt as if it were ripping something creative out of her. Although the anorexic part of the patient broadcast the idea that Mrs W had been contaminated by the therapy, she was also aware that her attack upon me resulted in the loss of an object that could help her to think: "The trouble is, when I lose my art, I lose my capacity to see." At the end of the session, when Mrs W spoke about her aunt describing the way food had dropped out of her mouth when she was small, I thought she was aware of the work we needed to do in chewing things over, and the work she needed to do in sucking and swallowing. However, she was alerting me to the pull towards this defiant and aggressive passivity. The risk was that in protest against the ending of the therapy, the meal we had worked on together could be allowed to fall out of her mouth as she refused to suck or to chew, leaving her starved of any psychic nutrition. Although as we worked towards the end of the therapy the developments gained came under renewed attack, they did not disappear. I also had to take account of the fact that while separation from the anorexic part of her mind made me feel we were making progress, the anorexic part of Mrs W's mind believed that the emergence of the oedipal situation and the loss of omnipotent control spelt disaster. As a result of the therapy she was, I believe, able to mourn the loss of her omnipotent defences and tolerate more separation from, and yet dependence upon, her objects.

Despite her reservations, after the individual therapy Mrs W was able to move on to group psychotherapy, where she continued her progress, with no further admissions to hospital. Her capacity to use the group and deepen her understanding of her difficulties was mirrored in her capacities: she maintained her marriage while at the same time developing her own career.

Discussion

If unsuccessfully treated, anorexia remains one of the most deadly illnesses in mental health: every year many patients die from chronic starvation. Patients often present themselves as being in control—indeed, they can be very good at persuading others that there is no problem. When working with patients who suffer from chronic anorexia, it is helpful to think of their minds as being dominated by a psychotic part that hates all appetites and denies the need for anything apart from relationships with objects they can control. The full extent of this psychotic hatred of reality and life may be concealed by another part, which often presents as being reasonable and in touch with reality. Indeed, these patients broadcast propaganda to undermine their own and others' sense of reality. The anorexic part of these patients is only interested in controlling their relationships and their objects, to the extent that they become lifeless. Patients who seem to be cooperating with therapy or treatment may, at the same time, be actively looking to control and starve the life out of the contact.

In the initial stage of Mrs W's therapy, her method of communication deprived me of the material I needed to understand her. This had the effect of pulling me into a position where the separation between us was denied in subtle ways. At the same time, I also grasped hold of material in an energetic way, rather like a starving man receiving his first bit of food. This allowed the patient to slip back into her anorexic state, and my interpretations were treated as if they were some sort of cold poison rather than nourishment.

After Mrs W's breakdown and admission to hospital, I was more mindful of my countertransference and subtle enactments, and this produced a dramatic change in her presentation. I became aware of the way I was being controlled by the envious and destructive anorexic part of her mind, which left the non-anorexic part of her mind starved of support. The narrative within the sessions increased, and the purpose of projective identification changed, as Mrs W became less concerned with controlling her object and denying separation. As a consequence I was given more material and room to think in sessions. This development was accompanied by the development of the non-anorexic part of the patient's mind that was looking for genuine contact with her therapist. However, although this was a positive step, I also had to understand the role that her passivity played in maintaining the starved psychic state. Her description of the way she had allowed food to fall out of her open mouth emphasized the fact that, at some point, the patient would become passive rather than do the work (of chewing or sucking) required for successful therapy. This seemed to me to represent not only an attack on any nourishment provided in the therapy, but also, I thought, a fear that I could not take her aggression. I think Mrs W thought that the process of chewing over what the therapy had meant for her, including her criticism, would be seen by me as attacking her rather than the work of the therapy. When I was not able to manage the countertransference, this resulted in a kind of force-feeding.

Over time I was able to interpret this behaviour rather than feel provoked into becoming over-active. I also had to take account of the fact that while separation from the anorexic part of her mind made me feel we were making progress, the anorexic part of Mrs W's mind believed that the emergence of the oedipal situation and the loss of omnipotent control spelt disaster. While the developments gained in therapy came under renewed attack as we worked towards the end of the therapy, they did not disappear. In fact, the patient was able to move onto group psychotherapy, where she continued her progress with no further admissions to hospital.

At the start of the therapy, the fragmented communication provoked me into becoming over-active. I also had to take account of the fact that separation from the anorexic part of her mind made me feel there was coherence and meaning in the communication, but this false therapeutic understanding was designed to prevent the emergence of genuine emotional contact between therapist and patient. Caper (1997) describes the need for the therapist to function like a parental couple, with the maternal aspect of the therapist being receptive to the patient's communications while the paternal aspect of the therapist prevents the projections from taking over and overwhelming the mother's mind.

Instead, I tried to tune in to the psychotic level of Mrs W's functioning. Over time, this led to a gathering of the transference into the therapeutic setting and a clarity and strength in her communications—a shift that allowed the emergence of fears that her object could not bear either her aggressiveness or her neediness. Gradually, by gathering in the communications to the transference, the patient was able to work through conflicts and anxieties concerning her internal world and her relationships and to separate herself from the influence of the anorexic internal structure. Although this was a frightening shift for Mrs W, as she was not sure whether her object could endure her aggressive attacks, we were eventually able to work through some of these anxieties, and she subsequently discovered capacities to make reparation in herself as well as resilience in her objects.

CHAPTER NINE

Hysteria: the erotic solution to psychological problems

The term "malignant hysteric" is used to describe patients who are often admitted to hospital under an MHA section, after gross acting out or abandoned and careless behaviour, which then pushes others to take responsibility for their lives. They can present with bizarre symptomatology, with psychotic phenomena and paranoid ideation; once on the ward, their presentation may quickly calm down, and within a few days they may be vying to run the ward groups or acting as therapists to other patients.

Patients may then argue that the mental health section needs to be removed and that they should be free to come and go from the ward as they please. They appear to be coherent, and the global picture of fragmentation and thought disorder has disappeared, so the Mental Health Review Tribunal usually agrees to remove the section. Subsequently, and in keeping with the patient's progress, a discharge plan is developed. Then suddenly, out of the blue, the patient acts out in a dramatic and frightening way, taking everyone by surprise, and posing a considerable clinical challenge to mental health staff.

The violence and suddenness of these patients' actions characteristically leads to a split in the staff team between those who see them as having a manipulative personality disorder and those who see them as "ill". These disagreements can affect the clinical team's capacity to function, and any discussion about the nature of the patients' condition is often contaminated by moralistic arguments regarding the authenticity of their presentation.

These patients often achieve a status of being "special", and the nature of their clinical problem pushes staff into adopting approaches that contradict normal practice.

One hospital manager, out of desperation, asked me to go to see a patient on a surgical ward. The patient, a 37-year-old woman, had been occupying a highly expensive and precious intensive therapy unit bed on a surgical unit for six months. She complained of having stomach pains that prevented her from eating, and consequently she had to be fed via intravenous drip. After numerous physical investigations, no organic cause of the pain was found. However, every time the ward team went to remove the intravenous drip, the patient would scream and then threaten staff with lawyers and litigation. She also refused to cooperate, during an assessment, with the liaison psychiatrist, becoming abusive and screaming at the psychiatrist that she "was not mad". The history was relevant because her adult life had broken down after she was jilted at the altar 15 years earlier. The patient regressed to behaving like a baby, refusing either to get out of bed or to leave her parents' house. From time to time and out of desperation, the parents would seek help from the GP. The patient would be admitted to a general hospital for investigation, only to be discharged several weeks later, with nothing physiologically abnormal reported.

During this particular hospital admission, the patient heard that a psychotherapist had been asked to look at her file. She said that this was against her wishes, and she demanded to see the hospital manager. During this meeting, the patient accused the manager of abuse and threatened to sue the hospital. After screaming and shouting at the manager, the patient got out of bed, removed the intravenous drip, and walked out of the hospital.

These patients often veer among a bewildering mixture of mental states, shifting from competent and rational to chaotic and fragmented, and this can evoke in staff a variety of responses, ranging from heroic wishes to save or cure them to rather moralistic accusations that the patients are manipulative or malingering. Relationships often become erotized, and cases of professional misconduct resulting from boundary violations are not uncommon. One patient I treated used to come into the outpatient waiting room in the middle of the afternoon wearing a feather boa and a ball gown. It looked as if we were meeting for a date rather than a psychotherapy session. Another patient I saw claimed to have had a sexual relationship with a psychiatrist many years earlier. She claimed that twenty years later the psychiatrist was still keeping in touch and monitoring the patient's mental state. She presented it to me as if the psychiatrist were terrified that the patient would disclose the affair and bring shame on himself and his family. In this way, guilt was used to control the psychiatrist and ensure that he never left her. This theme was also present in the therapy, as the patient demanded I offer her unconditional love and devotion in the face of her escalating self-harming behaviour. She believed I could never question the validity or therapeutic value of the therapy, as I could not face my own shortcomings or failings. In the transference, she believed I was like the psychiatrist whose narcissism interfered with his judgement and professionalism.

Britton (1999) describes the way hysterics try to actualize the Oedipus complex as a cure for their difficulties, rather than giving it up. They intrude into the parental couple's creativity, and their inability to separate from their parents' sexuality interferes with the development of their own sexual identity. He specifies imagination as a place in the child's mind where the parents' intercourse takes place when the child is not present, and room for its development comes into existence when the child can tolerate the idea of the parents' sexual relationship going on elsewhere—behind the bedroom door. It is the place where the object spends its time when the child is not actually present.

In therapeutic relationships, hysterics demand their therapists' exclusive love while attacking and undermining their relationship with others, including their internal relationship with psychoanalytic theory and practice. Patients in this state of mind can fill the consulting room with actions designed to saturate therapists' minds, inducing them into reacting, rather than thinking, and threatening with their erotized enactments the therapeutic setting and therapists' capacity to think. A particular problem can arise as any curiosity expressed by therapists or mental health professionals can be misinterpreted by patients as an erotic interest in them.

Case examples

Splits in the clinical team

A ward manager, a primary nurse, and an occupational therapist from an inpatient unit presented the case of Mr X.

Mr X was a 45-year-old man with multiple diagnoses, including schizophrenia and BPD. The ward manager said that the patient was splitting the nursing team, and he was worried that they could no longer manage him on the ward. He told the supervision group that there had been a pattern of care in relation to Mr X's previous admissions. Following a drug overdose, he would be placed on MHA section and admitted as an inpatient, but within days on the ward his mental state would settle down, and he would appeal against his mental health section. When his section was subsequently removed, he would leave the ward but return several hours later in an intoxicated state. Staff suspected Mr X supplied other patients with drugs, thus creating an atmosphere of excitement and mania on the ward.

Any discharge plan or referral to a rehabilitation hostel or therapeutic community was accompanied by a series of self-destructive or violent acts, which undermined the discharge plans. The ward manager confessed that they would eventually discharge Mr X, as the team had lost patience with his disruptive behaviour. After being discharged, he would start working the streets in order to support his drug habit, and his mental state would quickly deteriorate. He would then be re-admitted to the inpatient unit, via A&E, after taking a large overdose in a manic and euphoric state.

The ward manager said that Mr X had formally complained about several members of staff, and consequently the staff felt intimidated and angry. Mr X was charming towards the staff he liked but threatening, violent, and vindictive towards staff he did not. A division developed in the team between those who felt sympathetic to his difficulties and others who thought he was manipulative and bullying. The primary nurse said Mr X talked to her about a figure called John who was telling him to do self-destructive things. I asked her if she had noticed any pattern in Mr X's acting-out behaviour. She said that things seemed to get worse whenever she mentioned a discharge plan, as he would take an overdose or smash up his room. The primary nurse then said in a tentative way that she thought Mr X was quite attached to the ward.

History

Mr X's parents had both suffered from severe and enduring mental illness, and he was taken into care when he was very young, where his carers and foster parents abused him. When he left his foster home at the age of 15, he started taking drugs, and he supported his habit by working as a prostitute. At around this time he also developed an abusive relationship with a man called John, who supplied him with drugs in return for sex. In his case notes, it said that Mr X had a delusional belief that he was Jesus and a long-standing history of hypochondriacal anxieties and self-harm. On one occasion, he was sent to prison for grievous bodily harm.

I think it is helpful to think of hysterics as having psychotic and non-psychotic parts of their personality (Bion, 1957). The psychotic part is always ready to intrude into the non-psychotic part of the mind with offers of omnipotent, erotized solutions to painful psychological problems. These solutions are based on patients' ability to seduce the object by flattery into a false relationship that undermines the individual's relationship with reality. The psychotic part of the personality believes that erotized relationships offer the cure for all psychological pain and difficulties. Hysterical patients often throw themselves into sexualized relationships with little concern for themselves. The phantasy is that they can get rid of themselves in order to become whatever the object requires them to be. Having excited this erotized adoration in the object, patients demand endless reassurance that they are the apple of the object's eye. However, the object's reassurances are never trusted, because patients believe that the adoration has been achieved by a manipulation of reality. Their guilt about destructive attacks on reality is projected into another person, who is then accused of being seductive and false. When these narcissistic relationships break down, patients feel traumatized and accuse the object of betrayal, while regressing into a child-like state.

John represented a psychotic part of Mr X's mind that was always on hand to offer manic, sexualized solutions in order to deny Mr X's underlying difficulties. An example of this included the tendency to hand himself over to complete strangers with no thought for his safety or protection. Over time, this orgy of dissociated sadomasochistic sex led to a fragmentation of his ego. His way of abandoning himself to others in such an excited and reckless way pushed psychiatric services into a position where they had to step in and take responsibility.

Once on the ward, a split would develop between those members of staff who felt sympathetic to Mr X's behaviour and those who thought that he was trying to extort some form of secondary gain. He then encouraged the split by provoking conflict between the two groups. He complained to the sympathetic staff that other staff were uncaring and unprofessional, while treating the unsympathetic group with contempt. Staff opinion varied from a view that he was manipulative and "knew what he was doing" to the belief that he was being victimized by the psychotic voice called John. This split shifted the focus of attention away from the problem of Mr X's mind and the nature of his difficulties and onto the argument between the sympathetic and unsympathetic staff. The strength of feeling engendered meant that rather than coming together to discuss the patient as a whole, the staff team remained split, each half blaming the other.

Riesenberg-Malcolm (1996) highlights hysterics' primary relationship with an unavailable object. Because of the lack of an internal object to help them to bear and metabolize their experiences, hysterics have to evacuate unmanageable conflict or painful internal states into different relationships. Taking the form of actions and enactments with others, these evacuations externalize the conflict or painful internal situation. Exaggeration and hyperbole are used in order to get the communication through in a way that might overwhelm the object's capacity to think. Hysterics are continually threatened by fear of depressive breakdown followed by psychic fragmentation and collapse. They try to manage these anxieties by projecting different elements of their mental state into people around them in the external world.

Mr X unconsciously encouraged a split in the staff team in order to prevent the clinical picture from coming together. The reality was that the split in the team was an external manifestation of an internal split. He tried to portray himself as an integrated man capable of managing his own life—a presentation that denied his underlying fears of fragmentation and collapse. In reality, Mr X was closer in functioning to the level of a traumatized 3-year-old child than a grown man. The secondary gain was related to his wish to control the treatment situation, as he denied the real level of his dependence upon the mental health service while maintaining his position as a patient on an inpatient ward.

Despite the bad atmosphere on the ward, I was struck by the team's compassion and concern for Mr X in the face of considerable provocation. I thought the ward staff had done a good job, and in many ways they were victims of their own success. Mr X did not want to leave the ward, because he felt he had finally found a family that cared for him, despite his provocation and destructive behaviour.

Although on one level Mr X attacked and denied his anxiety and dependency, on another he needed staff to understand his anxieties about his mania and self-destructive behaviour and to survive his splitting and undermining of their functioning. Consequently, in the supervision group we discussed the need for the staff team to be reunited and helped to recover their professional objectivity and interest in the patient through thoughtful discussion. In this way, we were able to gather together different views and opinions held within the team. We also talked about the need for a multi-professional case conference in order to think through the clinical difficulties and future plans. This would enable the multidisciplinary team to share the problems together, while accepting that there were no magical solutions. In a case like this, where there is a likelihood that the patient will complain, it is important that senior managers understand some of the head-aches faced by the frontline clinical staff, who are unlikely to risk implementing unpopular care plans with patients who complain if they do not feel that management are supportive. For this reason, I thought it was important to invite senior management to the case conference, as they needed to hear about the clinical difficulties faced by staff.

I said to the primary nurse that it would be helpful for her to develop a long-term view of the patient's needs. I suggested she talk to Mr X about the way in which he tended to act out in order to eject his unmanageable feelings. She also needed to demonstrate to him that she understood that the likelihood of acting out would increase whenever the word "discharge" was mentioned to Mr X.

Several weeks after the case conference, the primary nurse presented the case of Mr X again, and the clinical picture had changed considerably. Even though the section had been removed, the patient remained on the ward for most of the time. He had stopped bringing drugs onto the ward, his self-harming behaviour was less frequent, and the difficulties between the staff team had lessened. The primary nurse reported that she had spent some time talking to the patient about his difficul-ties and worries about being discharged. She said that it had become clearer in her mind that he was actually very anxious about this, but they had begun a dialogue.

Over the next couple of months, a discharge plan was instigated in which it was agreed that there would be a hand-over period between the ward and the hostel to which Mr X was being transferred. The primary nurse escorted the patient to the hostel on several occasions and also met with the hostel staff to dis-cuss his care and some of the management challenges. Several months later, the patient transferred to the hostel, where he remained for several years.

Patients in disturbed states of mind fragment and project different parts of themselves into various parts of the mental health system, and this can lead to splits in teams and institutions. Supervision is an important part of the care system, as it helps staff to understand and work through their different feelings and perceptions about each patient. These patients require staff teams to comprehend that, although they act out and have perverse elements to their personality, they are also demonstrating the level of their functioning. They need staff teams to look at their functioning as a whole, rather than as individual instances of acting out or manipulation. If the team can take a long-term view of the patient's problems, they will better understand their need for containment and care over extended periods of time. It is helpful to think of this sort of patient as a member of the mental health services "family" who is likely to require admissions over many years. Indeed, when teams rush improvements or fail to acknowledge patients' underlying difficulties and level of disturbance, this can lead to an increase in acting out. Although patients who suffer from hysterical states of mind may deny the level of their dependency, they also need mental health teams to stay in touch with their underlying need and vulnerability.

Once a long-term containing structure has been established in which patients feel that the level of their disability has been taken on board by the clinical team, they may settle—and when and if they become "more calm", it will be possible to have a discussion with them about their difficulties.

Projection of guilt

A team from an acute admission ward presented the case of Mrs Y.

> Mrs Y was a 50-year-old patient with a diagnosis of post-traumatic stress disorder and substance misuse. A liaison psychiatrist described the patient as a repeat attender at A&E. She said Mrs Y's admission always took a similar pattern—she would phone the emergency services and tell them that she has taken a fatal overdose. She would arrive in A&E intoxicated and

escorted by several male police officers. As soon as the police officers left, she would become physically and verbally abusive; on many occasions, her behaviour and assaults on staff became so serious that staff would be forced to remove her from A&E. However, once removed, Mrs Y would take another overdose and report to a police station before being detained under mental health legislation and transferred to a psychiatric ward.

History

Both of Mrs Y's parents were drug addicts, and their relationship was characterized by violence and a preoccupation with their drug habit. The patient and her younger sister both suffered systematic violence and mistreatment. However, notwithstanding these difficulties, she managed to do well at school and to go on to university. Following university, and despite leading a chaotic lifestyle, Mrs Y held down a well-paid professional job. She had a long history of casual sexual relationships until she reached her late thirties, when she met a drug dealer. He introduced her to illicit drugs, they were married, and he moved into her flat. From time to time, she would be admitted to hospital following her husband's assaults. Despite the serious nature of these attacks, she always refused to press charges. However, eventually, after one serious assault, Mrs Y separated from her husband and subsequently divorced him.

Psychiatric history and contact with services

Soon after her divorce, Mrs Y presented to her GP, complaining of anxiety and depression. The GP prescribed Valium and antidepressants. According to the patient, the medication did not help her symptoms but, rather, began to interfere with her working life, and she lost her job. At this point she was referred to a psychiatrist, who was critical of the GP's prescription of Valium and put her on a different regime of medication. Mrs Y blamed the GP's prescription for the development of panic attacks and suicidal thoughts. Subsequently, she successfully sued the GP for prescribing the medication that had, she claimed, led to the loss of her employment.

The ward manager then told me about Mrs Y's most recent admission. Once on the ward, she developed an intense relationship with her male primary nurse. The ward manager said that she was concerned that the relationship was rather over-involved, although she did not feel it warranted re-allocating the primary nurse. She went on to say that some of the female staff noticed how Mrs Y would act in a seductive way towards her primary nurse, putting on make-up before seeing him and dressing in a provocative manner. The primary nurse dismissed the female staff members' concerns, claiming they were based on jealousy and their lack of understanding that the patient had been traumatized. The ward manager said that Mrs Y's behaviour became disruptive when her primary nurse was not on duty, but calmed down when he was there and able to give her one-to-one sessions. Staff tended to consider Mrs Y as the primary nurse's patient and referred all queries about the patient to him.

After Mrs Y had been on the ward for a number of weeks, her behaviour improved, and a discharge was planned. At the same time, her primary nurse was allocated another demanding patient, who required a great deal of attention. Mrs Y's behaviour deteriorated rapidly, and she became increasingly demanding. She then took a large overdose, demanding admission to the intensive care unit of a general hospital. While she was there, she asked whether her primary nurse could visit. When she was told that he had gone on holiday, she went into a withdrawn state, refusing to speak and eating very little. On her return to the mental health acute admission ward, she was told that her care had been transferred to a female primary nurse, and her discharge plan was still in place. After several aggressive outbursts Mrs Y discharged herself from the ward. Before she discharged herself, however, she contacted the hospital management to make a formal complaint, alleging that her original male primary nurse had had a sexual relationship with her while she was on the ward. He was suspended on the spot, and an investigation was started. Several months later, the hospital cleared the primary nurse of professional misconduct but insisted on regular supervision for his clinical work.

Mrs Y was identified with parents who were more interested in their need for stimulants and drugs as a manic cure for their problems than in the demands of their children. Thus, Mrs Y felt she was competing with the drugs and manic behaviour for her parents' attention. Despite this chaotic and neglectful environment, the patient managed to pass exams and worked hard in order to provide herself with a career. For a time, she was able keep her private life of drug-taking and promiscuity separate from her career and her work. However, when she married her drug-dealing husband, the split between her working and private life broke down. Her husband represented her reliance on manic mechanisms to avoid painful and depressing realities. She was also repeating the pattern of her traumatic childhood by marrying a man who turned to drugs and violence as a way of solving problems. When the split broke down, the manic and erotized defence attacked and undermined her healthy part, which had managed to work and establish a professional life. She struggled to face the loss of her self-esteem and the damage she had done to her professional career.

Brenman (1985) describes the false relationships, designed to deny the extent of their disturbance, that hysteric patients form with the object. Thus relationships are used to negate psychic truth rather than to face reality in the interests of development. Hysterics seduce the object into falling in love, as though this would provide the reassurance they require. Loving relationships are used to provide the illusion of cohesion and integration and avoid fears of disintegration and fragmentation. However, Brenman also points out that such patients are usually suspicious of these loving relationships, which they fear are false and prone to breaking down. This leads to on-going pressure on the object to provide more and more reassurance of their devotion and love—reassurances that are, however, often treated as valueless and false. Indeed, hysterics who seduce the object into being loving then accuse the object of being corrupt. In the therapeutic situation, hysterics often believe that therapists are trying to get patients to fall in love with them.

In her mind, Mrs Y seduced her GP into becoming an exciting and potent father figure who promised to take away difficult feelings about the collapse of her life with powerful drugs. Indeed, her desire to get rid of feelings of depression and loss about her situation led to her becoming addicted to erotized relationships with heroic figures as a cure. When this structure failed to provide the promised solution and threatened to break down, Mrs Y found another figure who offered even more powerful magical solutions: she replaced her GP and his failed magical solutions with the psychiatrist. Her guilt about her damaging addiction to omnipotent solutions was projected into the GP. In the transference, the GP turned into the abusive and neglectful father figure who offered her drugs rather than real support and interest as a solution to her problems. She then recruited the psychiatrist as an authority to back up her claim that she had been seduced, mistreated, and betrayed by the GP.

The scenario was repeated when the patient was admitted to an inpatient unit in a chaotic and disturbed state. She made the primary nurse believe that he was the one who was going to rescue her from her difficulties, provided he committed himself to her wholeheartedly.

We can see how Mrs Y tried to seduce her object into loving her, as she believed this would be the answer to her difficulties. She created an erotized, heroic rescuing phantasy in the GP, the psychiatrist, and the primary nurse, who were all seduced into believing that they were the solution to her difficulties. In one part of her mind, Mrs Y believed she would be cured by her saviour's romantic devotion, which would provide her with reassurance that she was the integrated, lovable object she craved to be: "I must be integrated and whole—look how much they love me." However, in another part of her mind, Mrs Y believed that this devotion was not to be trusted, because it had been achieved by seductiveness and flattery. Consequently, each was pushed to prove the extent of his devotion through his actions: the GP was encouraged to prescribe more and more tranquilizers; the psychiatrist had to go against his GP colleague; and the primary nurse got into an argument with other senior colleagues on the ward. It was as if Mrs Y were saying, "Look at how lovable I am: they would do anything for me—go beyond normal prescribing habits, criticize and undermine their colleagues, argue with their colleagues . . .". When the erotized relationships and solutions broke down, she accused the professionals of offering a false relationship, which, she believed, promised to cure her of her difficulties. Thus responsibility for the part of her mind that was always trying to seduce her into believing magical solutions was projected into an external object, who was then blamed for providing false treatment and cures.

The erotic countertransference

A psychotherapist presented the case of Ms Z, whom he saw in twice-weekly psychotherapy for two years.

> Although Ms Z, a disturbed 25-year-old woman, had done quite well at school and university, she led a double life: in the daytime she worked as a receptionist, and in the evenings she worked as a prostitute.

> During her childhood, Ms Z's parents had separated and re-united several times in the course of a stormy relationship. Her father gambled the family's money away, and the patient believed he had a sexual relationship with her younger sister. She complained that her older brother was taken seriously by the parents and had an academic career, while her mother called the patient a slut.

> In the early stages of the therapy, Ms Z described her relation-ship with a wealthy older man, who used to pay her to accom-pany him to parties. This activity interfered with her work, and from time to time a long weekend trip away with him interfered with her attendance at the first session of the week.

> In one of the early sessions, Ms Z talked about attending a party, and then she could not get up in the morning. She explained: "I am just spending time with my friends, dancing. I love dancing, and I just think, why not, I am fed up with having to struggle at work, what is the point? I did not go in today, because I am ill and I am not going to push myself." The therapist said that Ms Z wanted him to know that the therapeutic work was hard, and she was not sure she could manage it. However, despite the temptation for her to stay at the party of her mind, she had, in fact, turned up for her session.

> Ms Z said that she had been getting really angry with a man at work, because he was not doing his job. His job was to purchase

things, but he delayed purchasing, and then the price increased. The therapist said that he thought part of her was aware that she was not getting on with the job of paying for the therapy, and that somewhere she was aware that she might pay a higher cost at a later date. Ms Z said: "I'm fed up with having to work so hard. I just enjoy going to parties and meeting my friends and dancing." The therapist pointed out how at her parties she was free to become anyone she wanted to be and get away from her difficulties. Ms Z said: "I have met some lovely friends at the club, but I did begin to feel a bit bored when older men asked for my number." The therapist said that Ms Z was getting bored with these parties and knew that she needed to start committing to the therapy. The patient replied that the problem was that she loved buying clothes, and that she could earn as much in one night working at a party as she earned in one week in her office job.

Ms Z then told the therapist that she would not be at the session the following Monday, as she was going away on another long weekend, to earn some more money. The therapist said that Ms Z was throwing herself at these men in an excited way in the hope that she could get away from having to think seriously about herself. In this session, Ms Z projected anxiety into the therapist by talking about the way she abandoned herself to these older men. The therapist became agitated by the patient's destructive, manic, sexualized behaviour, while Ms Z remained calm and in control. The therapist followed the material but missed the significance of the mood. Ms Z was wrapped up in manic and excited sexual acting out, an acting out that pushed the therapist into feeling he must pursue the patient in order to rescue her from this destructive behaviour.

Britton (2003) described hysterical patients who interpret the therapist's interest and curiosity as love and erotic fascination and use material in the session to excite rescuing phantasies in the therapist. Therapists may be unaware of the way in which their interest is being encouraged by patients who present themselves as acting in a self-destructive or abandoned way in order to heighten the erotic sense of being pursued. In supervision, which is at some distance from the impact of projections, we are able to reflect on the session and see Ms Z's actions pulling the therapist into pursuing her in an attempt to stop her from prostituting herself. This dynamic was represented in the session by the story of the older men in the club who tried to get Ms Z's telephone number. In the session, the therapist was the one felt to be pursuing her, while she played hard to get.

The therapist's desire to help Ms Z by rescuing her from prostitution was correctly viewed by the patient as an omnipotent solution and a betrayal of the psychoanalytic method. This increased Ms Z's omnipotence, as in phantasy—and in subtle ways in reality—she was able to seduce whomever she wanted. The desire to convert the patient from being a prostitute to becoming a psychotherapy patient interfered with the usual therapeutic stance, providing, in turn, a hook for Ms Z to exploit her wish to triumph over the reality of the oedipal situation. After some time and on reflection, the therapist was able to separate himself from the erotic countertransference and re-establish the analytic setting. This led to the patient becoming depressed and a bit more worried about herself in an appropriate way.

Several months later, Ms Z started the session by saying, "I keep getting mixed up feelings when I'm here. I feel angry with my parents. Then when I leave I think, 'Oh well, everybody makes mistakes and everyone changes', and then at night I get so angry again. I think to myself that I despise my father. He would say, 'you are the one going down the wrong road', because I had a drink or anything. But he is allowed to do what he wants, get drunk, or tell me about his love life. I have to keep to his rules. I am not allowed to have an opinion or a mind of my own. I am never allowed a love life and not allowed to have relationships with boys. I am supposed to be like a robot."

Ms Z's parents divorced when she was 7 years old. "I have to listen to his divorce story over and over again, and I just want to tell him to shut up. But I don't, I just stand there and listen. Well, my father only wants to talk about the things he wants to talk about, and I have to control everything, I feel that I can't relax. I can't relax." Ms Z explained that she tried not to think too much, because every little thing made her paranoid. She described the way her father used to comment on her appearance, saying, "you are too fat", or "you are too this" or "too that". He also used to comment on things in an inappropriate way, "like saying that he could see that I was developing, or if I was wearing a tight top, he would say that he could see my breasts. He used to comment on my weight, the size of my nose, etc. Coming back from work, he would say that he could see how well my shirt fitted around my shape."

The therapist said that he thought Ms Z sometimes felt that he was pulled into making comments about her behaviour, for example, when she went to parties, but when he made these comments, the patient thought that his interest was inappropriate. Ms Z replied by saying that she thought the therapist had helped her to pull away from all of the messy relationships in her family. She went on to say, "but I did not like thinking about the way I try to fit in with my father. I don't think the therapy is going to cure me, but I do feel I'm like a caterpillar going to turn into a butterfly. I'm not cured, but I feel so much better." The therapist said that he thought Ms Z was aware of the way she could differentiate between different sorts of interests, and this gave her hope that she could change. Ms Z replied by describing a dream. In the dream, *she was holding a crying, traumatized baby, but she did not feel anything for the baby.* The therapist said he thought the traumatized baby was the part of her that was ignored and neglected when she was able to pull the therapist into inappropriate comments or interest. She said, "I don't want to absorb too much trauma. I don't want to think that's me in the dream, as it will ruin my confidence." The therapist said that Ms Z did not want to think about the way she became wrapped up and excited in the wrong sort of interest. Ms Z said that she used to feel empty and didn't have any opinions: "I was like an abused child that couldn't say no to anything."

In the case of Ms Z, we can see the influence of the psychotic part of her personality, which encouraged her to give herself over to others, as if this would provide her with a sense of value. In this way, she got rid of herself and her mind by becoming an exciting sexual object. In the session described above, we can see how the patient had changed and moved on as she realized that there were different sorts of relationships. We can also see the development of a non-psychotic part of her personality, which did not want that sort of sexualized therapy or therapist, but was looking for one who was genuinely interested in her as a person, not as a sexual object. This part genuinely appreciated the support provided by the therapy. However, to some extent we can see the way Ms Z could easily be pulled back into her fascination with her father and her wish to seduce him, even though she knew that this would lead to a restricted life in which he became her prisoner.

This progress in Ms Z's capacity to make genuine contact with the therapist and use the therapy improved and consolidated as the treatment went on. She gave up her work as a prostitute, took a job that made use of her education, and after the end of the individual therapy joined a group. Several years later, the group therapist informed me that the patient continued to make good use of the group.

Discussion

Hysterical patients can alternate dramatically between different mental states. They project different elements of their personality into different parts of their body and/or different external objects. They then try to control these projected aspects of themselves by splitting them and controlling the way they are seen by the object. The control over external objects is forcibly maintained, either through seductive invitations for the object to become a heroic rescuer, or via threats that the object will be viewed as someone who traumatizes the patient if the support the patient requires is not delivered. Different elements of the individual's emotional world are lodged in various relationships and/or different parts of the patient's body, which the patient tries to keep apart, fearing not only that any integration of the different views will lead to reprisals from the object, but that insight will present a picture of a personality that has been put together in a false way using stolen identities.

The reality is that these patients feel they have been constructed on a diabolical basis. One patient said she was terrified of having an epidural during childbirth, as she feared that all of her "madness" would pour out: "Everyone will see I'm a diabolical mess inside."

In the first clinical example, Mr X wanted to deny the extent of his underlying difficulties while keeping control of the treatment situation. He did this by splitting the team and seducing some staff while accusing others of mistreatment. Only once the staff split could be healed was progress made in Mr X's treatment.

These patients need clinical teams and services with clinicians who can see through the acting out, and the dramatic presentations, to the patient's difficulties and needs behind the drama. Although patients deny the reality of their underlying fragmentation, they are also terrified of being left alone with their difficulties, hence the fluctuation between "*la belle indifférence*" of their difficulties and the dramatic acting out, designed to force the object to continue caring for them.

Patients have often failed to establish a good and reliable relationship with the mother and the breast, and they turn to the father in an attempt to get help with their feelings of depression and despair. The internal object is, however, felt to be so damaged that they need the father to be a phallus that offers magical reparation rather than an ordinary penis that offers support and creative links (Birksted-Breen, 1996). Thus the relationship with the father is saturated with erotic desires. Although patients seek to be reassured that they are exciting and desirable, their fear is that this is a false relationship that will lead to betrayal and collapse, and that there is no object that could help them bear the pain of their underlying fragmentation. Mourning requires individuals to face feelings of guilt about the damage done to their good objects and to relinquish their reliance on psychotic processes that deny reality. These patients fear that mourning the loss of their omnipotence and reliance on psychotic solutions would lead to unbearable guilt, followed by fragmentation. Instead, guilt about the reliance on triumphant and manic defences is projected into an object, who is often accused of being false and guilty of betrayal.

In the second clinical example, Mrs Y accused various medical staff of misleading her as she failed to be cured by their magical and omnipotent solutions. This was, however, partly a projection of her guilt, as she seduced them into behaving like phallic father figures who, in her erotized transference, were offering her illicit love in place of authentic care.

In individual therapy, the erotic transference prevents the development of a serious and thoughtful relationship between therapist and patient. Change and progress can only come about once the therapist has found a way to understand the erotic countertransference. It is important for patients to feel that they are being looked after by individuals and teams who survive, both in phantasy and in reality, their attacks on the parental couple. Similarly, progress cannot be made in mental or physical health care settings until splits in the clinical team have been understood and addressed.

In the third clinical example, as the erotization of the therapeutic relationship diminished, it allowed authentic contact between Ms Z and the therapist to take place. Over time, this enabled Ms Z to separate herself from her tendency to erotization and seduction and to develop her capacities to relate with others in a genuine way, which, in turn, improved her ability to engage in relationships and work.

Conclusion

The mental health system has to contain and care for patients with profound psychological difficulties and often with fragile egos that are prone to fragmentation in the face of painful psychological anxieties and conflicts. Their minds may also be inhabited by destructive aspects of the personality that offer psychotic solutions to problems in order to avoid, rather than experience and bear, painful psychic realities. These various elements wrestle for control over the mind as patients' thinking veers between the psychotic and the non-psychotic parts of the personality.

Patients who suffer from a psychotic illness and/or personality disorder and find it hard to face the extent of their difficulties and suffering may withdraw from the world of shared emotional meaning and into a preoccupation with states of mind based on omnipotence and omniscience. Ordinary communication may be stripped of its symbolic value and capacity to convey emotional significance, creating a distance that leaves the mental health professional and/or the relatives feeling alienated and deprived of meaningful contact. The danger is that mental health professionals respond to this painful situation by becoming mechanistic in their thinking, leaving patients feeling that they are being cared for by professionals who respond to their attack on psychological meaning by keeping patients and their suffering at a distance. Professionals may unconsciously go along with patients' denial and rationalization by trying to understand them at a neurotic level and joining with them in a manic denial of serious problems. This avoids painful realities about the extent of the patients' damaged thinking, but the patients' sane part is then left to manage the psychotic part alone and without any psychological support. Alternatively, mental health professionals may try to crush the psychosis by attacking it with aggressive doses of medication designed to eradicate psychotic signs and symptoms. But even though psychotic states of mind are serious and may cause considerable suffering and pain to patients and their relatives, the psychosis cannot be eradicated completely, as it represents an aspect of the patient's mind. This is not to say that psychosis and its side-effects should not be treated—rather, that we may further persecute patients if we give the impression that an aspect of their mind is intolerable. The psychotic part of the personality may represent a destructive aspect of a patient's mind, but it needs to be thought about and accounted for. Mental health professionals need to try to tune in to the psychotic wavelength in order to support their patients' struggle with the psychotic aspects of the self.

Psychoanalytic supervision can help professionals to rediscover their imagination and their capacity to think about their patients' underlying emotional states and to renew their curiosity and enthusiasm for their work. Indeed, some participants have said that it reminded them of why they had come into mental health work in the first place.

Even patients diagnosed as suffering from a neurotic condition or personality disorder, though not obviously out of touch with reality, can demonstrate evidence of what psychotherapists may describe as psychotic thinking, which, though not necessarily psychotic from a psychiatric point of view, may nevertheless be based on omniscient and omnipotent ways of thinking and may be encapsulated in a neurotic symptom. Acutely disturbed individuals require mental health services to take action and intervene actively in their lives, even sometimes against their will. This is an important function of psychiatry and psychiatric practice, and a reluctance to act may be destructive and unhelpful. However, mental health services also need to take in and think about the meaning of their patients' symptoms, behaviours, and actions. In this book, I have argued that an absence of an adequate model for thinking about the effects of psychotic communications leaves professionals in danger of reacting to unconscious forces without understanding them.

The psychoanalytic model provides mental health professionals with a way of thinking about their patients that will help them to make sense of their experience; it also provides them with a language for describing psychological interactions that take place within therapeutic relationships and for articulating their experience of the patient in an objective and considered way. It helps professionals to see a different dimension of the patient through the countertransference and the therapeutic relationship by providing a model that builds bridges between the more traditional psychiatric model and the patient's personality and state of mind. It encourages professionals to be curious about their patients—about their functioning over time and in different areas of life.

The model is particularly helpful when thinking about psychotic levels of communication, and it can help put the missing emotional meaning back into concrete psychotic communications or acting out. It can improve clinicians' capacity to stay emotionally available and interested in the emotional life of their patients, even when this seems to be missing, and they may be able to listen out for moments of meaningful communication if the predominant form of communication is stripped of emotional meaning.

Patients who act out their disturbance in dramatic ways, who project into their bodies and/or develop sadomasochistic relationships with others, need mental health staff who are interested in understanding the nature of such communication. This does not necessarily mean that the patient either wants or could manage insight at this stage of the illness. However, most patients benefit from feeling that they have been understood, even if they become disturbed by insight in themselves.

Understanding that both psychological truth and psychological reality are essential to the development and maintenance of a healthy mind can help professionals to tolerate adverse aspects of the patient's personality and attacks on caring relationships.

Psychoanalytic theory provides a model for thinking about the way different elements of patients' minds have been projected into different parts of the mental health system, at times causing staff to act out as arguments develop between professionals or teams or individuals within teams. Bringing these projected elements together can help the team to deepen their understanding of patients and to heal splits between teams and individuals. Dynamic understanding is also helpful in thinking about patients in terms of their clinical management, because it helps staff to maximize the therapeutic aspects of their relationships with patients and therefore minimize the risk of non-therapeutic relationships.

Many patients' minds are dominated by internal figures that hate the emotional pain involved in life and offer, instead, murderous psychotic solutions. Patients may feel that these destructive states of mind are central to their ego's functioning, as the psychotic defences promise to protect them from the pain and anxiety involved in life. Psychoanalytic psychotherapy can help to identify the extent to which the patient is dominated by destructive internal structures and to differentiate various elements of the patient's internal world and enable professionals first to identify and then to support healthy and sane aspects of the patient's internal world. Over time and through the course of therapy, it can help patients to separate themselves from the influence of the pathological and destructive aspects of the self and show them that ordinary conflicts and emotions are bearable and necessary.

For some, it will not be possible to integrate these hostile internal structures, nor will they be able to get rid of them or deny their existence. They may, however, be able to separate from the influence of these destructive aspects of the personality—a process that inevitably involves relinquishing the influence of omnipotent defences against pain and anxiety and being exposed to the more ordinary, painful anxieties involved in living. They can also be exposed to feelings of humiliation and shame, which can in turn lead to negative therapeutic reactions and retreats into regressive states of mind and behaviour. Staff also need to be sensitive to patients' feelings of humiliation and shame. These feelings are often expressed through conflicts over power and authority.

Patients with chronic conditions may need long-term support for the healthy aspect of themselves, and this needs to be tolerated and understood by mental health professionals. It is also helpful to identify the way the forces within the patients' minds alternate between psychotic and non-psychotic parts of the personality. This is not a situation that is necessarily resolved forever, as the psychotic part of the personality may continue to influence patients' thinking, even in periods of remission. Indeed, it can return as part of a negative therapeutic reaction when patients are making progress, which can lead to a rapid deterioration of patients' functioning as the psychotic part of the personality returns to take up a central role in their mind.

Patients with a severe and enduring mental illness need to be helped to mourn the loss of their view of themselves as ideal and accept their illness or breakdown. This is a painful process, as it involves accepting their weaknesses and limitations, rather than fighting them. It is also means that the patient has to experience some depressive feelings of loss and guilt over unconscious attacks on good objects that have tried to help them—a difficult process that exposes them to fears of further of fragmentation and breakdown. Psychotherapists and other mental health professionals also have to help patients bear such anxieties about the fragility of mental health and depressive feelings of guilt about damage done to loved objects, including the self.

Ill patients can have a considerable effect on therapists by provoking them into acting out. Insight into the nature of patients' difficulties has to be understood and worked through by therapists before it can be interpreted to patients. This is particularly important when treating patients who are not able to bear the psychological pain involved until there is a feeling that they have the therapist's understanding and support. It is also true that enactments in the therapeutic relationship often need to be understood by therapists before issues underlying these enactments can be worked on in the therapy.

Working with people who have mental illness can be rewarding and enlightening, but it can also be frightening, boring, frustrating, anxiety provoking, and stupefying. Patients' communications and actions can have a disturbing effect on mental health professionals and can provoke them into reactions that are designed to control the patient's thinking or behaviour. Although at times actions taken by staff may be appropriate and necessary, they are likely also to be driven by a wish to control provocative or disturbing elements of the patient's mind. Ultimately, both staff and patients need to begin to understand these disruptive and destructive elements of their own thinking. Without this deeper understanding, there will be missed opportunities, as the underlying meaning of communication is lost, ignored, or crushed. Psychoanalysis offers a model for thinking about and providing meaning for the anxieties that drive us "out of our minds", and this can reduce the risk of thoughtless action.

Working therapeutically with patients with a severe and enduring mental illness needs time and support from psychiatric services colleagues. This enables therapists and patients to work through various stages of the therapy as they alternate between periods of engagement and of regression. It also takes time for the patient and the therapist to find a way of working together.

I have given many examples throughout of how I learned through my mistakes, as I have had time and support to learn about and think through my thinking and approach. Such resources and support are vital for the successful treatment of patients with long-standing difficulties. To some extent, therapists have to survive the attacks on the clinical efficacy of the treatment as well as tolerating the uncomfortable idea that the therapy may not work and/or may not be able to survive serious attacks on its efficacy and viability. This means that the patient has to share with the therapist some responsibility for the survival of the therapy.

I have found that supervision of frontline staff and the treatment of patients with a severe and enduring personality disorder complement one another. On the one hand, the experience of being with ill patients in psychoanalytic treatment gives therapists first-hand experience of the emotional field involved in the treatment of ill patients. I have also found that frontline staff are interested in psychoanalytic ideas, provided that they are supervised by someone who is well trained and has clinical experience of the cases they are treating and/or caring for. The constant struggle in therapy reminds therapists of the difficulties of the work, and this helps supervisors keep in touch with the limitations of understanding. On the other hand, examples of the dynamics and mental structures evident in the presentation of patients in the acute stage of illness provide a clear picture of the underlying psychopathology. Patients who are ill often provide clear and gross examples of psychopathology, as well as of the constant fluctuations between psychotic and non-psychotic parts of their personality, and discussions of these can help psychotherapists in their understanding of cases seen within the psychoanalytic setting. When conducting supervisions, it is also possible to see the sorts of defensive enactments patients manage to induce in staff. In many ways, it is true to say that both patients and mental health professionals defend themselves against emotionally painful contacts. It is, however, always important to remember that defences are both necessary and important: we all need to withdraw to a resting place, an "asylum", protected from the depression and guilt associated with insight on the one hand and paranoia or fragmentation on the other.

I have tried to demonstrate the clinical relevance of psychoanalytic thinking both in the treatment of patients with a serious and enduring mental illness and in the supervision of frontline mental health professionals. I have also tried to demonstrate the importance of the relationship between psychiatry and psychoanalytic psychotherapy in the treatment and care of patients. I believe that, in the treatment of ill patients, psychiatry needs psychoanalytic psychotherapy and psychoanalytic psychotherapy needs psychiatry. When they work well together, they act as the parents of the clinical setting, with the listening approach of psychotherapy complementing the objective and scientific approach of psychiatry. I believe that patients benefit from the two approaches working together in their best interests. This is the sort of container that can bear the madness the patient brings into the system. In many ways, this will enable mental health professionals to make room for madness in mental health.

REFERENCES

Alanen, Y. O. (1997). *Schizophrenia: Its Origins and Need-Adapted Treatment*. London: Karnac.

APA (2013). *Diagnostic and Statistical Manual of Mental Disorders, Fifth Edition (DSM–5)*. Washington, DC: American Psychiatric Association.

Bell, D. (2001). Who is killing what or whom? Some notes on the internal phenomenology of suicide. *Psychoanalytic Psychotherapy, 15*: 21–37.

Bell, D. (2013). *Mental Illness and Its Treatment Today*. London: Centre for Health and the Public Interest. Available at: http://chpi.org.uk/wp-content/uploads/2013/12/David-Bell-analysis-Mental-illness-and-its-treatment-today.pdf

Bell, D., & Novakovic, A. (2013). *Living on the Border: Psychotic Processes in the Individual, the Couple, and the Group*. London: Karnac.

Bick, E. (1968). The experience of the skin in early object-relations. *International Journal of Psychoanalysis, 49*: 484–486. Reprinted in: A. Briggs (Ed.), *Surviving Space: Papers on Infant Observation* (pp. 55–59). London: Karnac, 2002.

Bion, W. R. (1955). Language and the schizophrenic. In: M. Klein, P. Heimann, & R. E. Money-Kyrle (Eds.), *New Directions in Psychoanalysis* (pp. 220–239). London: Tavistock Publications. Reprinted London: Karnac, 1985.

Bion, W. R. (1957). Differentiation of the psychotic from the non-psychotic personalities. In: *Second Thoughts* (pp. 43–64). London: Heinemann, 1967.

Bion, W. R. (1958). On arrogance. In: *Second Thoughts* (pp. 86–92). London: Heinemann, 1967. Reprinted London: Karnac, 1984.

Bion, W. R. (1959). Attacks on linking. In: *Second Thoughts* (pp. 93–109). London: Heinemann, 1967. Reprinted London: Karnac, 1984.

Bion, W. R. (1962a). *Learning From Experience.* London: Heinemann. Reprinted London: Karnac, 1984.

Bion, W. R. (1962b). A theory of thinking. In: *Second Thoughts* (pp. 110–119). London: Heinemann, 1967. Reprinted London: Karnac, 1984.

Birksted-Breen, D. (1989). Working with an anorexic patient. *International Journal of Psychoanalysis, 70*: 30–40.

Birksted-Breen, D. (1996). Phallus, penis and mental space. *International Journal of Psychoanalysis, 61*: 39–52.

Brenman, E. (1985). Hysteria. *International Journal of Psychoanalysis, 66*: 423–432.

Britton, R. (1989). The missing link: Parental sexuality in the Oedipus complex. In R. Britton, M. Feldman, & E. O'Shaughnessy, *The Oedipus Complex Today: Clinical Implications* (pp. 83–101). London: Karnac.

Britton, R. (1999). Getting in on the act: The hysterical solution. *International Journal of Psychoanalysis, 80.*

Britton, R. (2003). *Sex, Death, and the Superego: Experiences in Psychoanalysis.* London: Karnac.

Caper, R. (1997). A mind of one's own. *International Journal of Psychoanalysis, 78* (2): 265–278.

Cartwright, D. (2002). *Psychoanalysis, Violence and Rage-Type Murder.* New York: Brunner-Routledge.

Cleckley, H. M. D. (1964). *The Mask of Sanity.* St Louis, MO: Mosby.

Evans, M. (1998). Problems in the management of borderline patients in in-patient settings. *Psychoanalytic Psychotherapy, 12*: 17–28.

Evans, M. (2014). "I'm Beyond Caring": A response to the Francis Report. The failure of social systems in health care to adequately support nurses and nursing in the clinical care of their patients. *Psychoanalytic Psychotherapy, 28* (2): 45–61. Reprinted in: D. Armstrong & M. Rustin (Eds.), *Social Defences Against Anxiety: Explorations in a Paradigm* (pp. 124–143). London: Karnac.

Evans, M., & Franks, V. (1997). Psychodynamic thinking as an aid to clear thinking. *Nursing Times, 93* (10): 50–52.

Fabricius, J. (1991). Running on the spot or can nursing really change? *Psychoanalytic Psychotherapy, 5* (2): 97–108.

Freud, S. (1895d). *Studies on Hysteria. Standard Edition, 2.*

Freud, S. (1911b). Formulations on the two principles of mental functioning. *Standard Edition, 12*: 215.

Freud, S. (1912b). The dynamics of transference. *Standard Edition, 12.*

Freud, S. (1923b). *The Ego and the Id. Standard Edition, 19*: 13–66.

Freud, S. (1924e). The loss of reality in neurosis and psychosis. *Standard Edition, 19*: 183–187.

Freud, S. (1950 [1892–1899]). *Extracts from the Fliess Papers. Standard Edition, 1.*

Garelick, A., & Lucas, R. (1996). The role of a psychosis workshop in general psychiatry training. *Psychiatric Bulletin, 20*: 425–429.

Goffman, G. (1968). *Asylums: Essays on the Social Situation of Mental Patients and Other Inmates.* New York: Anchor Books.

Hale, R., & Dhar, R. (2008). Flying a kite—observations on dual (and triple) diagnosis. *Criminal Behaviour and Mental Health, 18*: 145–152.

Heimann, P. (1950). On counter-transference. *International Journal of Psychoanalysis, 31*: 81–84.

Hinshelwood, R. D. (2002). Abusive help—helping abuse: The psychodynamic impact of severe personality disorder on caring institutions. *Criminal Behaviour and Mental Health, 12*: S20–30.

Hinshelwood, R. D. (2013). Schizophrenia, meaninglessness, and professional stress. In: D. Bell & A. Novakovic (Eds.), *Living on the Border.* London: Karnac.

Jackson, M. (1985). A psychoanalytical approach to the assessment of a psychotic patient. *Psychoanalytic Psychotherapy, 1* (2): 11–22.

Jaques, E. (1955). Social systems as a defence against persecutory and depressive anxiety. In: M. Klein, P. Heimann, & R. E. Money-Kyrle (Eds.), *New Directions in Psychoanalysis* (pp. 478–498). London: Tavistock Publications.

Jaspers, K. (1913). *General Psychopathology,* trans. J. Hoenig & M. W. Hamilton. Baltimore, MD: Johns Hopkins University Press, 1963.

Kernberg, O. F. (1975). *Borderline Conditions and Pathological Narcissism.* New York: Jason Aronson.

Kernberg, O. F. (2008). Transference focused psychotherapy: Overview and update. *International Journal of Psychoanalysis, 89*: 601–620.

Klein, M. (1929). Infantile anxiety-situations reflected in a work of art and in the creative impulse. In: *Love, Guilt and Reparation and Other Works 1921–1945* (pp. 210–218). London: Hogarth Press, 1975. Reprinted London: Karnac, 1992.

Klein, M. (1934). On criminality. In: *Love, Guilt and Reparation and Other Works 1921–1945* (pp. 258–262). London: Hogarth Press, 1975. Reprinted London: Karnac, 1992.

Klein, M. (1935). A contribution to the psychogenesis of manic-depressive states. In: *Love, Guilt and Reparation and Other Works 1921–1945* (pp. 106–127). London: Hogarth Press, 1975. Reprinted London: Karnac, 1992.

Klein, M. (1946). Notes on some schizoid mechanisms. In: *Envy and Gratitude and Other Works 1946–1963* (pp. 1–24). London: Hogarth Press, 1975. Reprinted London: Karnac, 1993.

Klein, M. (1957). Envy and gratitude. In: *Envy and Gratitude and Other Works 1946–1963* (pp. 175–176). London: Hogarth Press, 1975. Reprinted London: Karnac, 1993.

Lawrence, M. (2008). *The Anorexic Mind*. London: Karnac.

Lucas, R. (2003). Risk assessment in general psychiatry: A psychoanalytic perspective. In: R. Doctor (Ed.), *Dangerous Patients: A Psychodynamic Approach to Risk Assessment and Management*. London: Karnac.

Lucas, R. (2009a). Developing an exoskeleton. In: *The Psychotic Wavelength: A Psychoanalytic Perspective for Psychiatry* (pp. 235–246). Hove: Routledge.

Lucas, R. (2009b). Differentiating psychotic processes from psychotic disorders. In: *The Psychotic Wavelength: A Psychoanalytic Perspective for Psychiatry* (pp. 125–141). Hove: Routledge.

Lucas, R. (2009c). The Kleinian contribution to psychosis. In: *The Psychotic Wavelength: A Psychoanalytic Perspective for Psychiatry* (pp. 61–83). Hove: Routledge.

Lucas, R. (2009d). Psychotherapy and reducing the risk of suicide. In: *The Psychotic Wavelength: A Psychoanalytic Perspective for Psychiatry* (pp. 260–279). Hove: Routledge.

Lucas, R. (2009e). The psychotic wavelength. In: *The Psychotic Wavelength: A Psychoanalytic Perspective for Psychiatry* (pp. 142–156). Hove: Routledge.

Main, T. F. (1957). The ailment. *British Journal of Medical Psychology, 30*: 129–145.

Martindale, B. (2007). Psychodynamic contribution to early intervention psychosis. *Advances in Psychiatric Treatment, 13*: 34–42.

McCabe, R., Heath, C., Burns, T., & Priebe, S. (2002). Engagement of patients with psychosis in the consultation: Conversation analytic study. *British Medical Journal, 325* (7373): 1148–1151.

Menzies, I. E. P. (1960). The functioning of social systems as a defence against anxiety: A report on a study of the nursing service of a general hospital. *Human Relations, 13*. Reprinted in: I. E. P. Menzies Lyth, *Containing Anxiety in Institutions: Selected Essays, Vol. 1*. London: Free Association Books, 1988.

Minne, C. (2003). Psychoanalytic aspects to the risk containment of dangerous patients treated in high-security hospital. In: R. Doctor (Ed.), *Dangerous Patients: A Psychodynamic Approach to Risk Assessment and Management* (pp. 67–78). London: Karnac.

Minne, C. (2007). Psychoanalytic aspects to the risk containment of dangerous patients treated in high security. In: D. Morgan & S. Ruszczynski (Eds.), *Lectures on Violence, Perversion and Delinquency: The Portman Papers* (pp. 59–82). London: Karnac.

Minne, C. (2008). The dreaded and dreading patient and therapist. In: J. Gordon & G. Kirtchuk (Eds.), *Psychic Assaults and Frightened Clinicians: Countertransference in Forensic Settings* (pp. 27–40). London: Karnac.

Money-Kyrle, R. (1956). Normal counter-transference and some of its deviations. *International Journal of Psychoanalysis, 37*: 360–366. Reprinted in: *The Collected Papers of Roger Money-Kyrle* (pp. 330–342), ed. D. Meltzer & E. O'Shaughnessy. Strath Tay: Clunie Press, 1978.

Money-Kyrle, R. E. (1969). The fear of insanity. In: *The Collected Papers of Roger Money-Kyrle* (pp. 434–441), ed. D. Meltzer & E. O'Shaughnessy. Strath Tay: Clunie Press, 1978.

O'Shaughnessy, E. (1992). Psychosis: Not thinking in a bizarre world. In: R. Anderson (Ed.), *Clinical Lectures on Klein and Bion* (pp. 85–98). London: Routledge.

O'Shaughnessy, E. (1999). Relating to the super-ego. *International Journal of Psychoanalysis, 80*: 861–870. Reprinted in: *Inquiries in Psychoanalysis: Collected Papers of Edna O'Shaughnessy*, ed. R. Rusbridger. Hove: Routledge, 2015.

Patrick, M., Hobson, R., Castle, D., Howard, R., & Maughan, B. (1994). Personality disorder and the mental representation of early experience. *Developmental Psychopathology, 6*: 617–633.

Rey, H. (1994). *Universals of Psychoanalysis in the Treatment of Psychotic and Borderline States*. London: Free Association Books.

Riesenberg-Malcolm, R. (1996). "How can we know the dancer from the dance?" Hyperbole in hysteria. *International Journal of Psychoanalysis, 77*: 679–688.

Riviere, J. (1936). A contribution to the analysis of the negative therapeutic reaction. *International Journal of Psychoanalysis, 17*: 304–320.

Rosenfeld, H. (1971). A clinical approach to the psychoanalytic theory of the life and the death instincts: An investigation of the aggressive aspects of narcissism. *International Journal of Psychoanalysis, 52*: 169–178.

Ruszczynski, S. (2008). Thoughts from consulting in secure settings: Do forensic institutions need psychotherapy? In: J. Gordon & G. Kirtchuk (Eds.), *Psychic Assaults and Frightened Clinicians: Countertransference in Forensic Settings* (pp. 85–95). London: Karnac.

Segal, H. (1950). Some aspects of the analysis of a schizophrenic. *International Journal of Psychoanalysis, 31*: 268–278. Reprinted in: M. H. Lader (Ed.), *Studies of Schizophrenia*. Ashford: Headley Bros.

Segal, H. (1957). Notes on symbol formation. In: *The Work of Hanna Segal: A Kleinian Approach to Clinical Practice* (pp. 49–65). New York: Jason Aronson, 1981.

Segal, H. (1977). Countertransference. In: *The Work of Hanna Segal: A Kleinian Approach to Clinical Practice* (pp. 81–87). New York: Jason Aronson, 1981.

Sohn, L. (1985a). Anorexic and bulimic states of mind in the psycho-analytic treatment of anorexic/bulimic patients and psychotic patients. *Psychoanalytic Psychotherapy, 1*: 49–56.

Sohn, L. (1985b). Narcissistic organization, projective identification, and the formation of the identificate. *International Journal of Psychoanalysis*, 66: 201–213.

Sohn, L. (1997). Unprovoked assaults: Making sense of apparently random violence. In D. Bell (Ed.), *Reason and Passion: A Celebration of the Work of Hannah Segal*. London: Duckworth.

Steiner, J. (1985). Turning a blind eye: The cover-up for Oedipus. *International Journal of Psychoanalysis*, 12: 161–172.

Steiner, J. (1990). The retreat from truth to omnipotence in Sophocles' *Oedipus at Colonus*. *International Review of Psycho-Analysis*, 17: 227–237.

Steiner, J. (1993a). *Psychic Retreats: Pathological Organizations of the Personality in Psychotic, Neurotic and Borderline Patients*. London: Routledge.

Steiner, J. (1993b). Two types of pathological organizations, In: *Psychic Retreats: Pathological Organisations of the Personality in Psychotic, Neurotic and Borderline Patients* (pp. 116–130). London: Routledge.

Steiner, J. (2011). The numbing feeling of reality. *Psychoanalytic Quarterly*, 80: 73–89.

Steiner, J., & Harland, R. (2011). Experimenting with groups in a locked general psychiatric ward. *Psychoanalytic Psychotherapy*, 25 (1): 16–27.

Steinhausen, H.-C. (2002). The outcome of anorexia nervosa in the 20th century. *American Journal of Psychiatry*, 159 (8): 1284–1293.

Taylor-Thomas, C., & Lucas, R. (2006). Consideration of the role of psychotherapy in reducing the risk of suicide in affective disorders—a case study. *Psychoanalytic Psychotherapy*, 20: 218–234.

WHO (1992). *The ICD–10 Classification of Mental and Behavioural Disorders*. Geneva: World Health Organization.

Williams, G. (1997). Reflections on some dynamics of eating disorders: No-entry defences and foreign bodies. *International Journal of Psychoanalysis*, 78: 927–942.

Yakeley, J. (2010a). Psychopathy. In: S. Frosh (Ed.), *Working with Violence: A Contemporary Psychoanalytic Approach* (pp. 41–55). London: Palgrave Macmillan.

Yakeley, J. (2010b). Psychoanalytic approach to risk assessment. In: S. Frosh (Ed.), *Working with Violence: A Contemporary Psychoanalytic Approach* (pp. 97–113). London: Palgrave Macmillan.

INDEX

211

in the United States
Taylor Publisher Services